Don't be a stranger to the delicious world of fresh food.

Your mother may have taught you to sniff melons, press the breastbone of chicken, and look for hard apples at the grocer's. But today's markets offer a dazzling array of exotic new fruits, vegetables, seafood, meats, and poultry. Small enough for your pocket or purse, *Le Gette's Guide to Fresh Food Shopping* is your guide through the aisles, the food handbook that can tell you:

- what variety of apples to look for
- how to test kumquats and passion fruit for freshness
- which variety of onion is best for your needs
- what good truffles look like
- how to buy venison, rabbit, frog's legs, and other gourmet meats
- the characteristics of over fifty different fresh and salt water fish
- which cooking methods are best for the many cuts of meat

And much, much more in . . .

Le Gette's Guide to *FRESH FOOD SHOPPING*

Also by Bernard Le Gette

Le Gette's Calorie Encyclopedia

Published by
WARNER BOOKS

Le Gette's Guide to FRESH FOOD SHOPPING

Bernard Le Gette

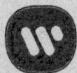

WARNER BOOKS

A Warner Communications Company

Warner Books, Inc.
666 Fifth Avenue
New York, N.Y. 10103

Ⓦ A Warner Communications Company

Printed in the United States of America

First Printing: July, 1985

10 9 8 7 6 5 4 3 2 1

TABLE OF CONTENTS

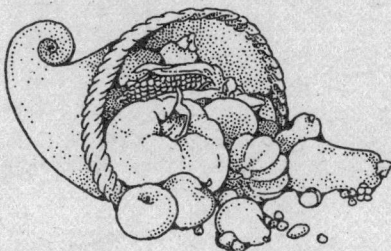

INTRODUCTION

There has never been so much food. As recently as the thirties chicken was a somewhat fancy dish—when you wanted to have that little something extra for holidays or guests. And it hasn't been twenty years since one dared to have anything besides turkey on the big holidays. The reason, of course, is that there wasn't that much available. Ducks, geese, and Cornish hens were all rather exotic meals, most people had never even tasted fresh artichokes or chanterelles,

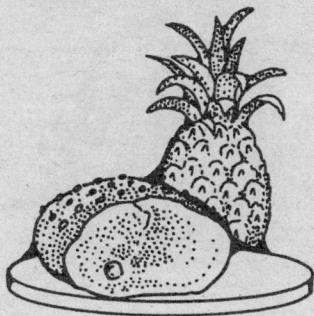

and abalone was an expression of disbelief.

But now? A gourmet shop in every other supermarket, butcher shops with freezers full of strange birds, and produce markets with vegetables you can't pronounce and fruits with fur.

It used to be easy. Whoever bought the vegetables bought them every day, had only five to pick from, and sooner or later even the slowest would catch on. But with the growth of canned, boxed and frozen packaging, everyone lost touch with the look and smell and feel of good fresh food. The overwhelming bulk of shoppers now have no idea which melons

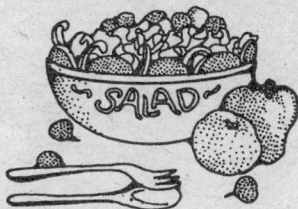

are the ripest, what you do with endive, or even how to peel a garlic. And that's the easy part. The wealth of fresh, delectable, nourishing, and even low-calorie food at our fingertips is out of reach if you don't know what it is, or how to buy it, or what to do with it when you get it home. Everyone's interested. Healthful natural food has graduated from its emaciated days of yore to become the preoccupation of us all.

But we can't all go back to Grandpa's farm to help him harvest peas. The farms are large and far away, the harvesting is done by machines, and besides, the peas are available all year at the corner store.

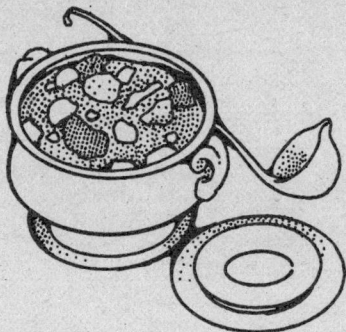

But even peas, though they're the oldest of all vegetables, remain a mystery to a lot of people. And it isn't a simple case of ignorance.

With all the people I spoke to about choosing and storing food—grocers, butchers, fishermen, and farmers—and all the books, lists, and government charts I researched, it became clear that there is a lot of confusion. Some things like fish and endive change their names through different regions, and the disagreements over things like whether or not loose pineapple leaves mean anything can bring people close to blows. The jury is still out on that one, by the way.

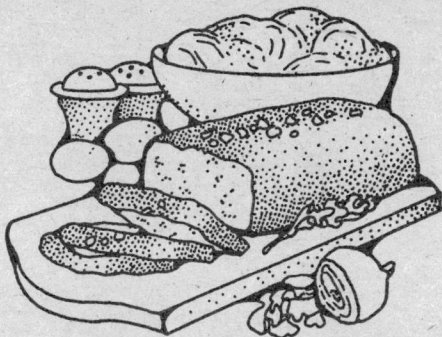

So what I've tried to do is boil down the information to the things most everybody agreed on. I've tried to keep everything as brief and clear as possible, so that if you wanted to you could bring this book to the market and actually be able to use it while you shop. In any case, it stores very well at room temperature and keeps indefinitely.

Fruit

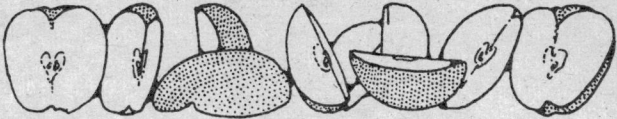

APPLE

Though everyone divides apples into two main categories—eating and cooking—there is no agreement on which apples belong in which group, except that Red Delicious, the most popular (41 percent of sales), is for eating, and that Spitzenbergen and York Imperial are for cooking. Otherwise, it's up to you. There are thousands of varieties; here are some of the most popular:

Cortland—large, dark red with red stripes, slightly tart, tender.
Crab—very small, bright red, round, extremely tart.

3

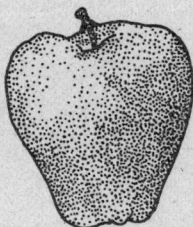

Empire—medium, red with stripes, sweet.
Golden Delicious—large, creamy green to golden yellow, sweet.
Granny Smith—medium large, rich green, crunchy, juicy, tart.
Gravenstein—medium, red, juicy, spicy, tart.
Jonathan—small, bright red, tart.
Macoun—medium, red with yellow striping, tasty.
McIntosh—medium, green blushed with red, slightly tart.
Newtown Pippin—medium to large, light green, round, crisp, tart.
Red Delicious—medium, deep red, sometimes striped, elongated, five knobs on blossom end, mildly sweet.

Rhode Island Greening—medium, yellow, crisp, slightly tart.

Rome Beauty—medium, bright red or green with red, juicy, aromatic, tart.

Stayman—medium, red, sometimes a little yellow, tart, keeps well.

Winesap—small, dark red, round, very crisp, juicy, slightly tart.

York Imperial—medium, red, round, crisp, juicy, tart.

Season: October–June, except year round for both Red and Golden Delicious.

Look for: firm, smooth, rich color.

Avoid: tender, bruised.

Store: refrigerate in a plastic bag; in quantity, keep cool, dark, dry, well ventilated.

Tips: ripen, individually wrapped in tissue paper, in a dark place like a drawer.

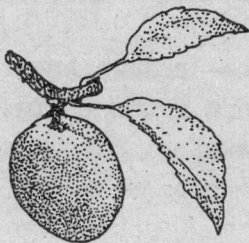

APRICOT

Season: June–August.
Look for: round, minor indentation, rich yellow with slight blush.
Avoid: hard, bruised, dull.
Store: ripen at room temperature in paper bag.

BANANA

Season: all year.
Store: ripen at room temperature, then refrigerate.

Yellow
Look for: firm, unblemished, greenish tip.
Avoid: soft, bruised, blackened.

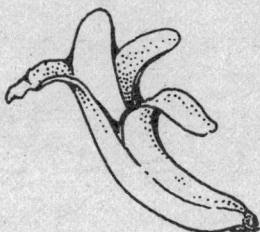

Red
Look for: firm, minor bruises okay.
Avoid: bruised excessively, black.

Plantain
Look for: firm, deep green.
Avoid: soft, bruised excessively.
Tips: • buy green, then ripen to yellow or black.
• they are always eaten cooked either like a vegetable or plain with lemon juice.
• peel in cold running water to avoid staining hands.

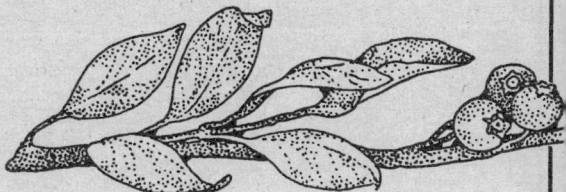

BLACKBERRY

Season: summer, early autumn.

Look for: plump, shiny, dark.

Avoid: soft, bruised, moldy, seepage, any red at all.

Store: remove decayed and bruised berries, wrap, and refrigerate.

Tip: do not wash berries until you are ready to use them.

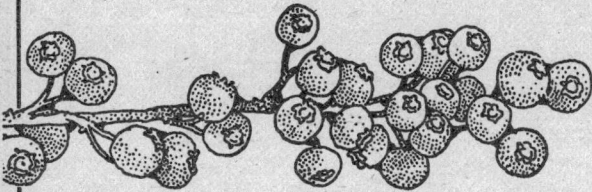

BLUEBERRY

Season: May–September.
Look for: plump, firm, frosty-looking skin.
Avoid: soft, bruised, moldy, small, and green.
Store: remove decayed and bruised berries, wrap, and refrigerate.
Tip: do not wash berries until you are ready to use them.

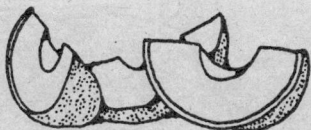

CANTALOUPE

Season: June–August.

Look for: heavy, fragrant; stem cavity smooth and yields to pressure; thick, coarse netting, yellow or gold in between.

Avoid: green or bright yellow, soft spots, cracked.

Store: ripen at room temperature, then refrigerate in closed bag.

Tip: do not cut before ripe.

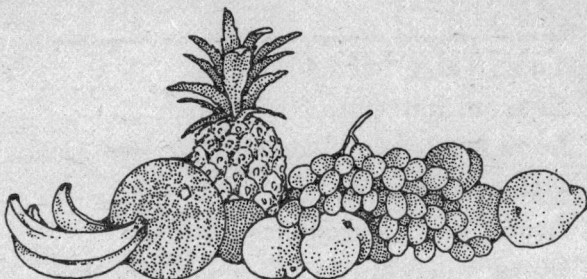

CARAMBOLA (STAR FRUIT)

Description: yellow, elongated, five ridges connected at the center.

Season: October–December.

Look for: pale to deep yellow (ridges dark on the edge), plump.

Avoid: mushy, bruised, blemished.

Store: ripen at room temperature in a paper bag, then refrigerate.

CASABA MELON

Season: June–October.

Look for: heavy, golden yellow; stem cavity yields to pressure.

Avoid: dark, soft spots.

Store: ripen at room temperature, then refrigerate in closed bag.

Tip: do not cut before ripe.

CHERIMOYA

Description: armored, purplish green, tastes like a litchi.

Season: winter.

Look for: plump, dull green, tender.

Avoid: bruised, mushy, brown.

Store: brown slightly at room temperature, then refrigerate no more than two days.

Tip: do not eat the seeds.

CHERRY

Season: June–August.
Look for: dark, plump, firm, shiny, with green stems attached.
Avoid: shriveled, mushy, mold, soft spots.
Store: refrigerate wrapped.

COCONUT

Season: all year.
Look for: heavy; sloshing sound when shaken.
Avoid: cracks, wet, moldy, lightweight.
Store: before opening, about a month or two at room temperature; after opening, about a week in refrigerator.
Tips: to open, pierce eyes with ice pick, drain liquid (good for drinking), place in 350° oven 20 minutes, tap with hammer.

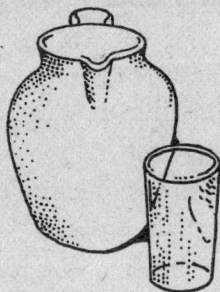

CRANBERRY

Season: October–December.
Look for: plump, shiny hard, nice red.
Avoid: soft, leaky, bruised.
Store: refrigerate or freeze.
Tips: sort out soft and wet berries before use.

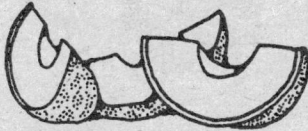

CRENSHAW MELON

Description: yellow, blotched with green, acorn shape, as big as your head.

Season: June–September.

Look for: fragrant, heavy; stem end yields to pressure.

Avoid: soft spots, dull, hard, cracked.

Store: ripen at room temperature, then refrigerate in closed bag.

Tip: do not cut before ripe.

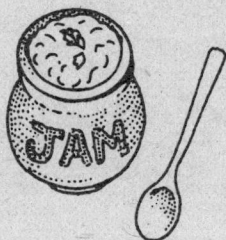

CURRANT

Description: small translucent berry (red, white or black), pleasingly sour; not to be confused with dried raisins.

Season: summer–fall.

Look for: plump, rich color.

Avoid: rust, soft, bruised, moldy.

Store: remove decayed and bruised berries, wrap, and refrigerate.

Tip: especially good with ham, venison, and in salads.

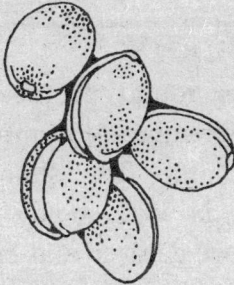

DATE

Season: August–November.
Look for: soft, plump, shiny smooth.
Avoid: hard, shriveled, sticky, or fermented.
Store: refrigerate wrapped.
Tip: fresh dates are pleasantly light, not nearly as heavy and sweet as the dried dates we usually eat.

ELDERBERRY

Description: round, purple-black berry.
Season: September–November.
Look for: plump, firm, shiny.
Avoid: soft, bruised, moldy.
Store: remove decayed and bruised berries, wrap, and refrigerate.
Tip: elderberry blossoms can be eaten deep fried.

FIG

Varieties: Black Mission (purple), Green Mission, Smyrna.
Season: June; August–October (the second season is better).
Look for: tender, fragrant.
Avoid: mushy, sour smell, breaks in skin.
Store: refrigerate no more than two days.

GALIA MELON

Description: like a large rusty-colored cantaloupe with coarser netting; from Israel.

Season: August–October.

Look for: heavy, firm; stem end yields to gentle pressure.

Avoid: soft spots, cracks.

Store: ripen at room temperature, then refrigerate in a closed bag.

Tip: do not cut before ripe.

GOOSEBERRY

Description: berry looks like a big green grape with white stripes.

Season: fall.

Look for: fleshy, firm.

Avoid: rust, soft, bruised, moldy.

Store: remove decayed and bruised berries, refrigerate, and wrap.

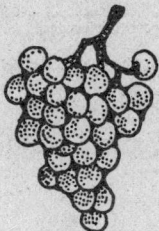

GRAPE

Cardinal—bright red, seeds, firm, sweet.

Concord—purple, seeds, strong rich flavor, juicy.

Emperor—red, seeds, mild.

Muscat—yellowy green, seeds, sweet, fragrant.

Red Seedless—dark red, mild.

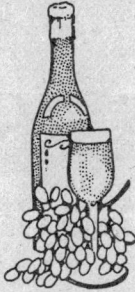

Thompson Seedless—light green, sweet, the most popular.
Tokay—firm flesh, keeps well.

Season: August–October.
Look for: frosty appearance, plump, slightly green flexible stems; red grapes should be mostly red, green grapes slightly yellow.
Avoid: bruised, dry, whitish, loose from stems, dry brown stems.
Store: refrigerate wrapped and unwashed.
Tip: wash just before eating to lengthen storage time.

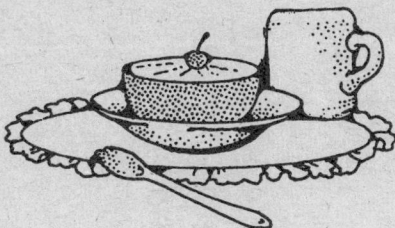

GRAPEFRUIT

Season: all year.
Look for: heavy, round, firm, bright color, smooth.
Avoid: lightweight, rough, wrinkled, soft, brown.
Store: at room temperature or refrigerated.
Tip: thin skin means more juice, though not necessarily more taste.

GUAVA

Description: looks like a yellow apple.
Season: June–August.
Look for: light yellow.

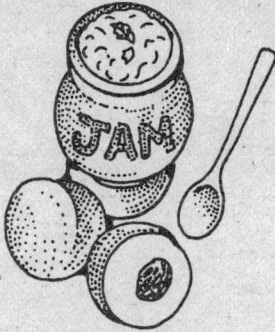

Avoid: brown spots, mushy.
Store: in refrigerator.
Tip: very high in vitamin C.

HONEYDEW MELON

Season: June–September.
Look for: heavy, slightly fragrant, sticky smooth surface; stem cavity yields to pressure; creamy color.
Avoid: soft spots, dull, hard, smooth, under 6-inch diameter.
Store: ripen at room temperature, then refrigerate in closed bag.
Tip: do not cut before ripe.

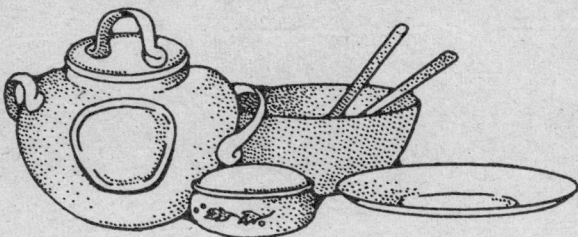

KIWI FRUIT

Description: hairy brown grenade, tastes somewhat like a cross between banana and grape.

Season: all year.

Look for: plump, tender.

Avoid: bruised, withered, hard, or mushy.

Store: ripen at room temperature, then refrigerate.

Tip: slightly fragrant when ripe; peel before eating.

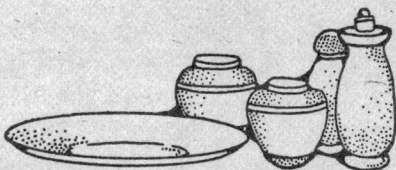

KUMQUAT

Description: tiny, oblong, orange-like skin.

Season: October–December.

Look for: firm, bright, shiny.

Avoid: soft, mold, dull skin or leaves.

Store: refrigerate wrapped.

Tip: eat the entire fruit; the sweet skin and sour pulp balance each other.

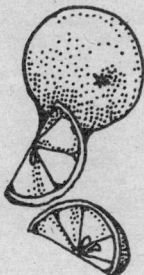

LEMON/LIME

The differences between these two close cousins are very subtle. The usual lime is the Persian. The famous Key Lime is a smaller yellow variety local to Florida.

Season: all year.
Look for: heavy, plump, firm, bright color, smooth.
Avoid: dull or rough skin, soft, marks, mold; lemons that are dark or hard are old and dried out.
Store: refrigerate.

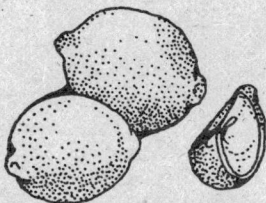

Tips: • roll firmly on counter several times at room temperature for more juice.
• juice retards browning of cut apples, bananas, pears, and avocados.

LITCHI
Description: walnut size; brown, scaly shell covering a soft white center.
Season: winter.
Look for: crispy feel to shell.
Avoid: dried out or mushy shell.
Store: refrigerate.
Tip: do not eat pit.

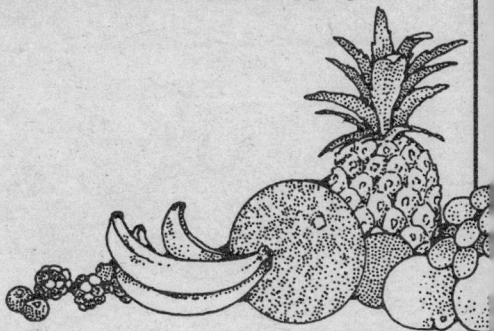

LOGANBERRY

Description: a dark red cross between a blackberry and a raspberry.

Season: June–August.

Look for: plump, shiny, tender.

Avoid: bruised, mushy, seepage.

Store: remove decayed and bruised berries, wrap, and refrigerate.

LOQUAT

Description: yellow-orange relative of the apple.

Season: March–June.

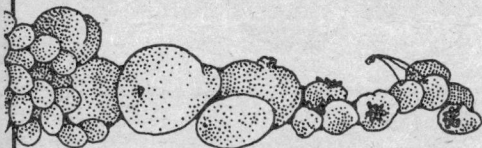

Look for: bright, tender.
Avoid: soft spots, bruises.
Store: in cool, dry, ventilated place.

MANGO

Season: May–September is best, though all year is possible.
Look for: tender, plump, smooth, orange-yellow; pleasant, fresh fragrance.
Avoid: green, hard, mushy, bruised.
Store: ripen at room temperature, then refrigerate.
Tip: serve very cold.

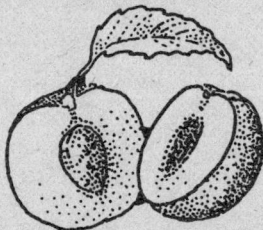

NECTARINE
Season: July–September.
Look for: slightly firm, yellow or even cream, fragrant.
Avoid: green, mushy, bruised.
Store: ripen at room temperature in paper bag, then refrigerate.

ORANGE

Seville
Description: a bitter orange used for marmalade, sauces, and salads.
Season: February–March.
Look for: heavy, firm.
Avoid: bruised, soft, mold.
Store: refrigerate in a paper bag.

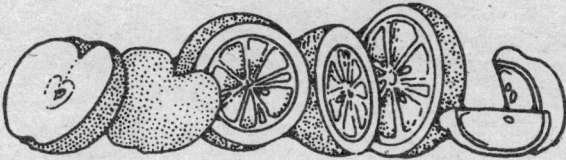

Sweet
Blood—varied colors from orange to red, sweet to tart.
Jaffa—late winter juice orange from Israel.
Navel—circular mark on stem end, thick skin, easy to peel and section.
Valencia—the most popular juice orange.
Season: all year.
Look for: heavy, firm.
Avoid: lightweight, soft, mold, very rough skin.
Store: refrigerate.

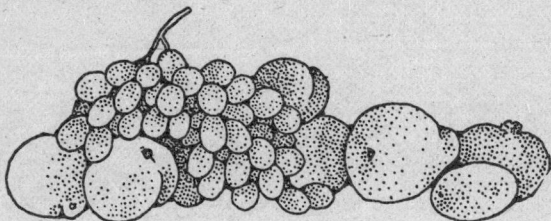

PAPAYA

Season: April–June.

Look for: firm, some yellow (the more yellow the better).

Avoid: soft, all green, pebbling, bruised.

Store: ripen (till all yellow) in paper bag, then refrigerate.

Tip: scoop out seeds, eat chilled with dash of lemon or lime juice.

PASSION FRUIT

Description: a purple, wrinkled egg with a sweet, juicy pulp.

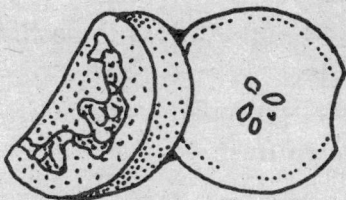

Season: July–November.
Look for: dark, dusty, irregular skin, tender.
Avoid: pale, hard or mushy, bruised, very smooth.
Store: ripen at room temperature in a paper bag, then refrigerate.

PEACH

Clingstone—pit adheres to flesh; mostly for canning.
Freestone—pit separates easily from flesh; mostly eaten fresh.

Season: July–September.
Look for: slightly firm, yellow or even cream, fragrant
Avoid: green, mushy, bruised.
Store: ripen at room temperature in paper bag, then refrigerate.

PEAR

There are about 5,000 varieties and probably all good. Here are some of the most popular:

Anjou—medium, ovoid, light to yellowish green, more gold when ripe.

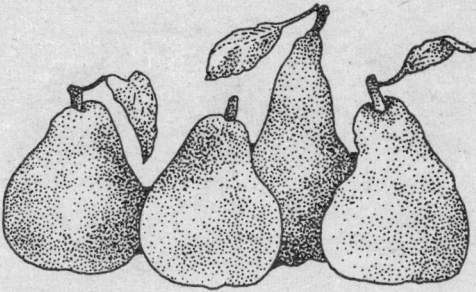

Bartlett—medium, pear-shaped, green turning to yellow or gold, or red-orange.
Bosc—medium, dull yellow green to brown, firmer texture.
Chinese—large, oval, light brown.
Comice—medium, stubby, pear-shaped, light to yellow green, the finest of pears.
Seckel—small, almost round, light green to brown.

Season: August–February.
Look for: characteristic color, firm, large.
Avoid: very hard or soft, bruised, blemished.
Store: refrigerate.
Tip: ripen, individually wrapped in tissue paper, in a dark place like a drawer.

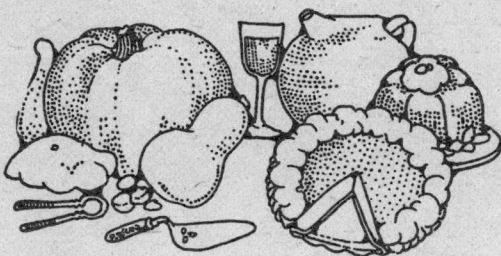

PERSIMMON

Description: yellow-red, like an elongated tomato, four-leaf cap.

Season: September–December.

Look for: waxy shine, golden orange, tender.

Avoid: hard, green, blemished, cracked.

Store: ripen in a paper bag at room temperature, then refrigerate.

Tips: taste before eating; should be sweet.

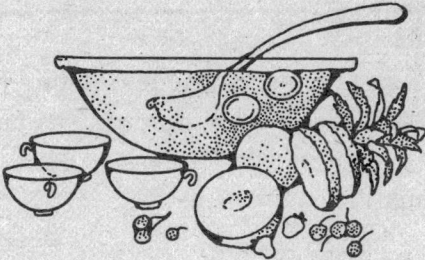

PINEAPPLE

Season: all year.
Look for: fragrant, golden or red-brown, short crown, heavy.
Avoid: dull color, very green, dried, unpleasant odor, soft, brown crowns.
Store: eat within two days.

PLUM

There are many varieties, among them Damson, El Dorado, Empress, Greenage, Purple, Red, and Santa Rosa. All are delicious.

Season: May–October.
Look for: smooth frosty skin, rich color (green plums should be slightly yellow), tender.
Avoid: hard or mushy, brown, cracked, leaky.
Store: ripen at room temperature, then refrigerate.

POMEGRANATE

Season: September–December.
Look for: heavy, large, bright.
Avoid: lightweight, small, shriveled, dull, cracked.
Store: refrigerate.

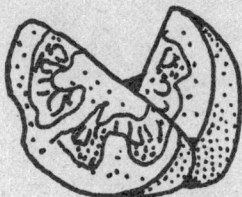

Tips: • the juice will stain clothes.
   • to get to the fruit, cut into the stem
     end and break fruit into halves, cut
     these in half, pull rind from seed
     sacs.

PRICKLY PEAR

Description: red or green cactus (spines
removed) with pink flesh.
Season: September–February.
Look for: firm, red turning green or green
turning yellow.
Avoid: mushy, brown, dried out.
Store: ripen at room temperature, then
refrigerate.

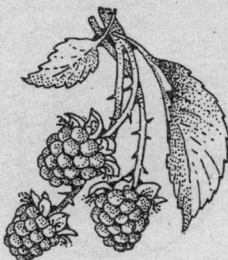

QUINCE

Description: a lumpy yellow relative of the apple, somewhat tart.

Season: October–December.

Look for: firm, yellowing.

Avoid: soft or hard, very green, bruised.

Store: ripen in a paper bag at room temperature, then refrigerate.

Tip: great in marmalade and jam because of natural pectin.

RASPBERRY

Season: June–August.

Look for: plump, tender, caps gone and hollow.

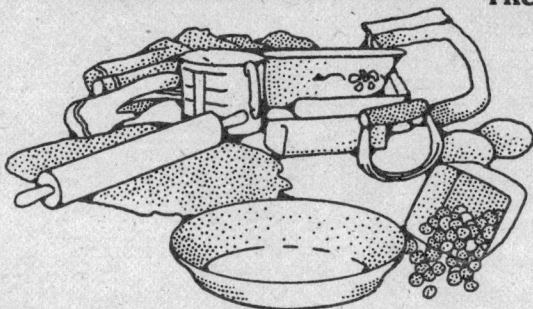

Avoid: bruised, mushy, seepage, large areas lacking color.

Store: remove decayed and bruised berries, wrap, and refrigerate.

Tips: • there is also a smaller and juicier autumn crop.

• do not wash berries until you are ready to use them.

RHUBARB

Season: March–August.

Look for: crisp straight stalks, red or pink, bright.

Avoid: oversized, wilted, scrawny stalks.

Store: refrigerate.

Tip: the leaves are poisonous; eat the stalks cooked with sugar.

41

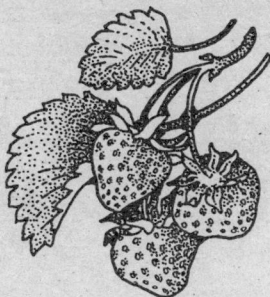

STRAWBERRY

Season: June–August.

Look for: bright, firm, green caps attached.

Avoid: bruised, mushy, seepage, large areas lacking color.

Store: remove decayed and bruised berries, wrap, and refrigerate.

Tip: do not wash berries until you are ready to use them.

TANGERINE

Description: similar to Clementine, Tangelo, Minneola, and Mandarin, all hybrids from oranges.

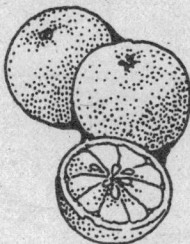

Season: December–February.
Look for: heavy, bright color.
Avoid: lightweight, pale, mold, very soft.
Store: refrigerate.

UGLI FRUIT
Description: a misshapen, yellow-green, ugly, delicious grapefruit.
Season: January–April.
Look for: heavy, round, rich color.
Avoid: soft, brown.
Store: refrigerate.
Tips: the ugli is eaten like and is sweeter than grapefruit.

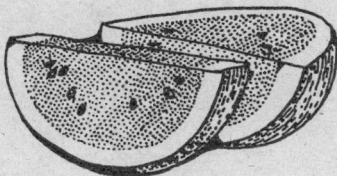

WATERMELON

Season: June–August.

Look for: heavy, firm; underside slightly creamy color; flesh should be deep, rich red.

Avoid: white streaks, soft spots, cracks, mealy flesh.

Store: refrigerate; keeps longer uncut.

Tip: the seeds are tasty toasted.

Vegetables

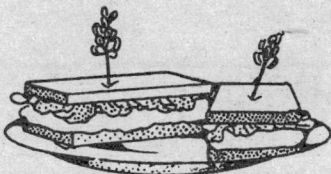

ALFALFA

Description: fine creamy white sprouts with green tips, in bunches.
Season: all year.
Look for: crisp, green and white.
Avoid: soggy, wilted, yellow.
Store: refrigerate.

ARTICHOKE

Season: all year; March–May best.
Look for: heavy, firm, tightly closed, green ("winter-kissed" are slightly darker).
Avoid: brown, spreading leaves.
Store: refrigerate.
Tip: before cooking cut spine tip from each leaf with scissors.

ARUGULA

Description: looks like watercress, slightly nutty flavor, becomes bitter when old.
Season: May–October.
Look for: rich green, fairly crisp.
Avoid: yellow, overgrown, wilted.
Store: refrigerate wrapped.
Tip: wash by immersing, not with running water, to avoid bruising the leaves.

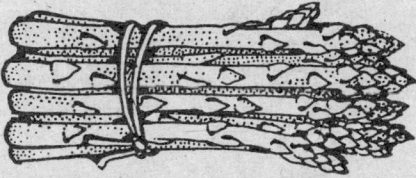

ASPARAGUS

Season: March–June.

Look for: tight tips, firm, crisp, smooth, straight, green extending well down the stalk.

Avoid: flat or opening tips, vertical ridges.

Store: refrigerate wrapped.

Tips: • eat either raw or cooked.
  • to trim, rather than cutting off the ends, grab each end and bend the asparagus until it snaps, which will be at just the right place.

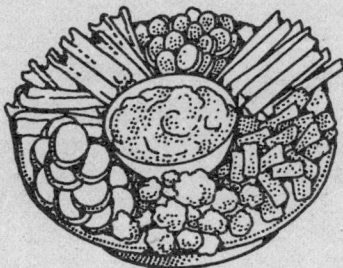

AVOCADO
California—large, slightly watery.
Florida—large, slightly watery.
Fuerte—pear-shaped, succulent.
Hass—thick, pebbled, purple-black skin, oily, perhaps the best.

Season: January–May.
Look for: firm to slightly tender.
Avoid: hard or mushy, bruised.
Store: ripen in paper bag, then refrigerate.
Tip: to keep an unused half from turning black, leave the pit in and cover.

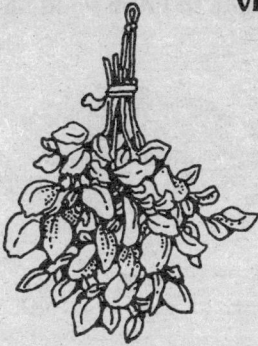

BASIL

Often called Sweet Basil (green), but includes Opal (purple), Lemon, Lettuce Leaf, and Miniature.

Look for: rich green color.

Avoid: yellow, rust, buds.

Store: refrigerate in slightly damp paper.

Tip: wash only before eating.

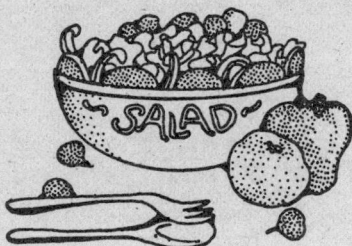

BEANS, Green

Season: all year, best in summer.

Look for: young crisp pods that snap, a velvet surface, bright color.

Avoid: flabby, wilted, thick pods, shriveled ends, seeds visible through pods, rust, overgrown.

Store: refrigerate wrapped.

BEAN SPROUTS

Season: all year.

Look for: rich creamy color, somewhat crisp.

Avoid: wilted, dull.

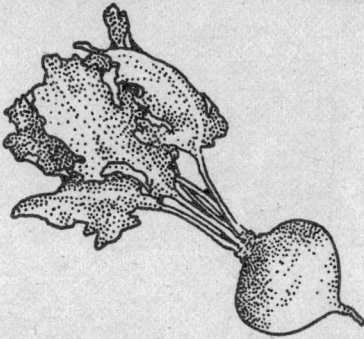

Store: refrigerate.

Tip: don't buy too much and eat right away for best flavor.

BEET

Season: all year.

Look for: small, firm, smooth, round; the greens should be fresh looking.

Avoid: wilted greens, soft wet spots, elongation.

Store: refrigerate wrapped.

Tips: • the greens can be cooked or used in salads.

   • clean beet stain off hands with salt.

53

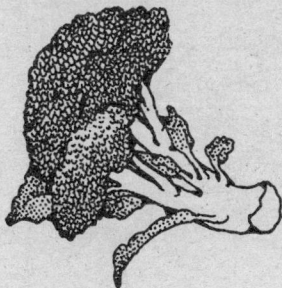

BEET GREENS

Season: all year.
Look for: crisp, rich green.
Avoid: wilted, yellow, rot.
Store: refrigerate wrapped.
Tip: cook like spinach or use in salad.

BROCCOLI

Season: all year.
Look for: firm stalks, dark color, compact.
Avoid: spreading top, yellow, wilted.
Store: refrigerate wrapped.

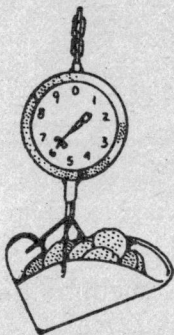

BRUSSELS SPROUT

Season: October–February.
Look for: bright green, firm, tight.
Avoid: yellow, soft, wilted or loose leaves.
Store: refrigerate wrapped.
Tips: cook no more than 7–8 minutes.

CABBAGE

Green—light green to white, smooth leaves, best for cole slaw.

Savoy—light to medium green, crinkled leaves.

Red—maroon leaves.

They can be used interchangeably.

Season: all year.
Look for: heavy, compact, rich color.
Avoid: wilted, yellow.
Store: refrigerate wrapped.

CARROT

Season: all year.
Look for: shiny, smooth, firm and crisp, fresh-looking greens.
Avoid: green skin, sprouting.
Store: refrigerate wrapped.

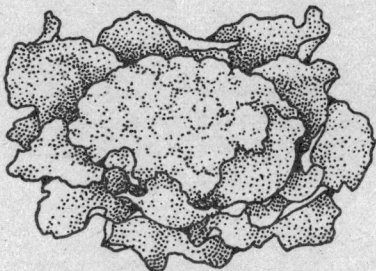

Tip: sweaty packaged carrots indicate they have been sitting around too long.

CAULIFLOWER

Season: all year, September–November best.
Look for: compact, heavy, solid, fresh green leaves.
Avoid: discoloration, spreading, rust.
Store: refrigerate wrapped.
Tip: soak in cold salted water to remove insects.

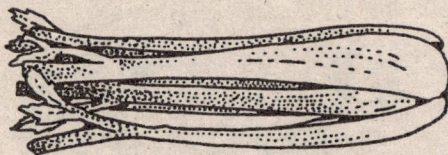

CELERIAC (CELERY ROOT)

Description: a bulbous root, brown with white inside.

Season: winter.

Look for: firm, medium size.

Avoid: soft.

Store: in a cool, dry, dark, well-ventilated place.

Tip: slice and peel before cooking.

CELERY

Season: all year.

Look for: crisp, heavy, very firm, fresh leaves.

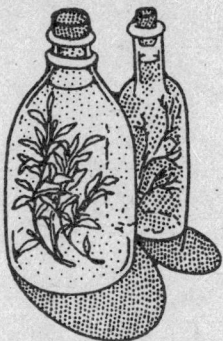

Avoid: limp, soft, overgrown, rust.
Store: refrigerate wrapped.
Tip: if it becomes limp, soak in ice-cold water a few minutes.

CHERVIL
Description: looks like a flat, feathery parsley, more subtle taste.
Season: all year.
Look for: bright green, crisp, fresh-looking, pleasant smell.
Avoid: wilted, dry, brown.
Store: refrigerate in damp towel.

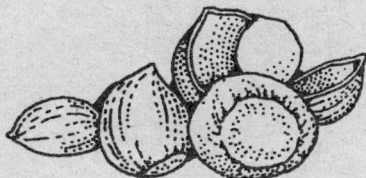

CHESTNUT

Season: October–December.
Look for: heavy, bright brown, shiny, big.
Avoid: dull, lightweight, shriveled.
Store: in a cool, dry, well-ventilated place.
Tip: before boiling or roasting, cut a cross in tip to avoid bursting.

CHINESE CABBAGE

There are many varieties, some of them called Bak Choy.

Season: all year.
Look for: crisp, fat stems.

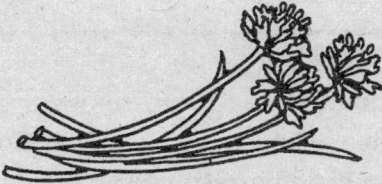

Avoid: soft, wilted, gray.
Store: refrigerate wrapped.
Tips: • use raw in salads.
      • when cooking sauté or stir fry
       briefly for best flavor.

CHIVES
Description: looks like long round grass
but is a delicate-tasting onion.
Season: all year.
Look for: good rich green, crisp.
Avoid: wilted, yellow, soggy.
Store: refrigerate or freeze.

61

COLLARDS

Description: broad, green, smoky-textured leaves; usually known as one of the Greens; it is a non-heading relative of the cabbage.
Season: November–March.
Look for: crisp, pleasant green, plump stem.
Avoid: wilted, yellow, holes, or eaten.
Store: refrigerate wrapped.

CORIANDER (CHINESE PARSLEY)

Description: looks like pale, flat-leafed parsley.
Season: all year.
Look for: crisp leaves, good color, pungent odor.
Avoid: wilted, dry, yellow or brown, unpleasant odor.
Store: refrigerate wrapped.

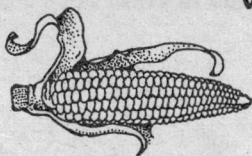

CORN

There are many varieties, but your local kind picked fresh is the best you will taste.

Season: summer. Though available all year, it loses its wonderful texture and flavor within a couple of days of being picked, but can be found fresh during the warm months in any area of the country.

Look for: green husks, fresh silk, fat, even kernels.

Avoid: yellow, wilted, or dry husks; brown, shriveled, or irregular kernels.

Store: refrigerate, eat as quickly as possible.

Tip: if you are told not to peel back the husk a bit to look inside, you probably shouldn't buy the corn.

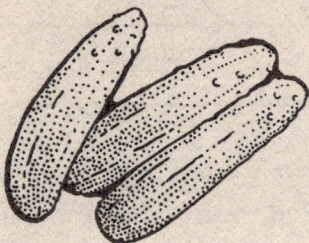

CUCUMBER

~~Kirby~~—small, plump, less likely to be waxed.
~~Seedless~~—very long, usually waxed or sealed.

Season: all year.
Look for: firm, rich green, unwaxed in the summer.
Avoid: white or yellow, soft, wet spots.
Store: refrigerate wrapped.
Tips: the wax is a preservative, which should be washed off with a brush.

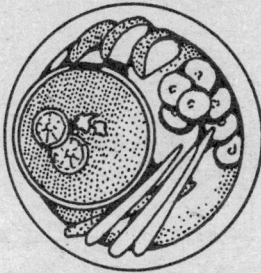

DANDELION GREENS

Description: a small spiky-leafed green plant.

Season: all year.

Look for: bright green, somewhat crisp, root still attached.

Avoid: wilted, yellow, gray.

Store: refrigerate wrapped.

Tip: great in salads.

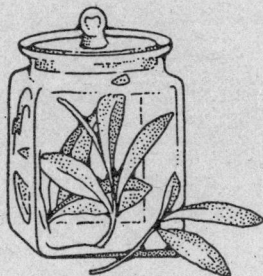

DOCK (SORREL)

Description: a small, broad, pointed green leaf with stem, at once fresh and sour.

Season: all year.

Look for: bright green, some crispness.

Avoid: yellow, wilted; hard, stringy stems; oversized leaves.

Store: refrigerate wrapped.

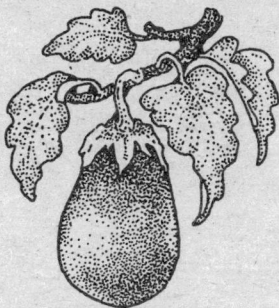

EGGPLANT

Chinese—purple, long, and slender.
Purple—large, always available; the smaller Italian are harder to find.
White—large, round, usually fall.
Yellow—small, round, usually fall.

Season: all year.
Look for: heavy, firm, shiny, rich color.
Avoid: cracked, dark spots, bruised.
Store: refrigerate wrapped.
Tips: • to get moisture out, salt after slicing.
   • An oval dimple at the blossom end (female) is said to indicate meatier flesh and fewer seeds than a round dimple (male).

67

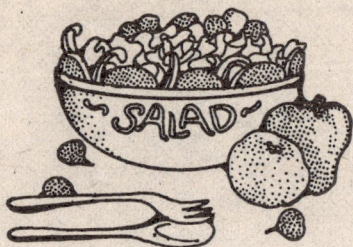

ENDIVE

There are a variety of plants called endive and chicory, with a matching variety of expert opinions on which plants belong to which categories. Just to give you an idea of the confusion, the most popular endive is called escarole. The reason for all this is that different regions of the country, not to mention other countries, have different names for them. Here's my list:

Belgian Endive—a trim white stalk about 6 inches long, mildly bitter, usually eaten raw in salads.
Look for: tight, firm, cream color with yellow tips.

Avoid: brown or green, spreading of leaves.
Store: refrigerate wrapped and keep it in the dark.

Chicory—looks like lettuce with curled and pointed narrow leaves; eaten raw in salads.
Look for: crisp, small heads.
Avoid: wilted, brown.
Store: refrigerate wrapped.

Escarole—looks like a small lettuce, splayed rather than round, white on the bottom, green on top; eaten raw in salads.
Look for: crisp, small heads.
Avoid: wilted, brown.
Store: refrigerate wrapped.

Radicchio—looks like a red-and-white lettuce, bitter, eaten raw or slightly cooked in salads.
Look for: crisp, small heads.
Avoid: wilted, brown.
Store: refrigerate wrapped.
Season: all year.

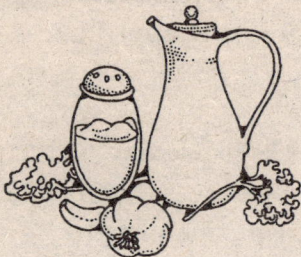

FENNEL

Description: cream to light green bulb with feathery leaves on stalk.

Season: November–March.

Look for: bright green, with a thick white base when still attached.

Avoid: bruised, wilted, split.

Store: refrigerate wrapped.

Tip: anise flavor, good raw in salads or cooked in soup, roasts.

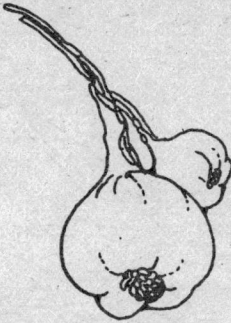

GARLIC

Season: all year.
Look for: heavy, solid, unbroken.
Avoid: brown spots, sprouting, soft.
Store: whole, in a cool, dry, ventilated place, not in the refrigerator.
Tip: to peel easily, press down sharply with flat of large knife or blanch in boiling water 20 seconds and slice off the root end when cool enough and the skins will slip away.

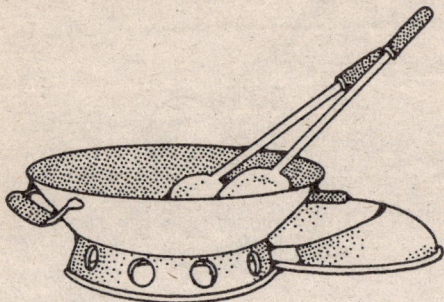

GINGER

Description: a hard, misshapen, knobby, tan root.

Season: all year.

Look for: smooth, not too many knobs or branches, large sections.

Avoid: musty, shriveled, too many knobs.

Store: refrigerate or freeze.

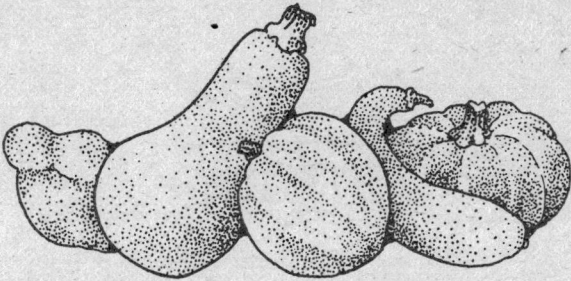

GOURD
Chayote—green, tear-drop shaped, 4-inch maximum; tastes like water chestnut.
Chinese Okra—dark green, ribbed, 6–8 inches; slice off the ribs before cooking; similar to zucchini.
Hercules War Club—light green, long and slender, 6-inch maximum eating size, something like zucchini.

Season: March–October.
Look for: heavy, firm, bright color.
Avoid: dull, soft spots, flabby, mold.
Store: cool, dry place.

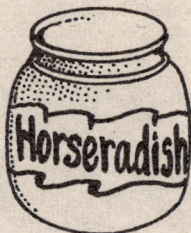

HORSERADISH

Description: a brown, gnarled root, hot, usually grated.
Season: all year.
Look for: firm, crisp, fat.
Avoid: shriveled, soft spots, sprouting.
Store: refrigerate.

JERUSALEM ARTICHOKE

Description: looks like a cross between ginger and a potato; crunchy, mildly sweet.
Season: all year.
Look for: firm, crisp, plump.

74

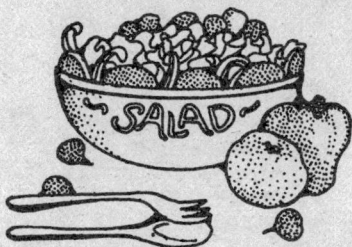

Avoid: soft, sprouting, shriveled.
Store: in a cool, dark, dry, well-ventilated place.
Tips: • may be eaten raw or cooked.
   • wash and scrub well before cooking and peel afterward when it's easier.

JICAMA
Description: Mexican water chestnut, potato-like, sweet, not starchy.
Season: all year.
Look for: firm.
Avoid: soft, cracked, mold.
Tip: usually peeled, sliced, and eaten raw.

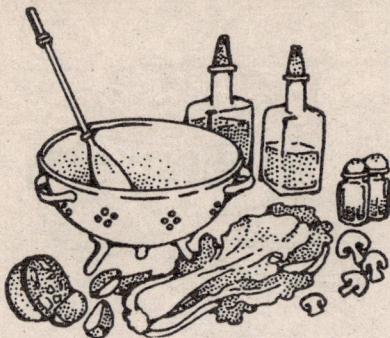

KALE

Description: green, fluffy-edged leaves on a stem.

Season: November–March.

Look for: crisp, rich green.

Avoid: yellow, wilted, rot.

Store: refrigerate or freeze.

KOHLRABI

Description: a firm, pale green bulb; looks like a small, alien cabbage; tastes something like turnip but more delicate.

Season: November–March.

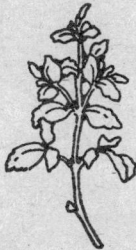

Look for: firm, bright, crisp.
Avoid: yellow, mushy.
Store: refrigerate.

LAMB'S LETTUCE (MACHE)
Description: clover-like but larger.
Season: September–February.
Look for: crisp, rich green with a touch of blue.
Avoid: wilted, yellow, dry.
Store: refrigerate wrapped.
Tip: best raw in salads.

77

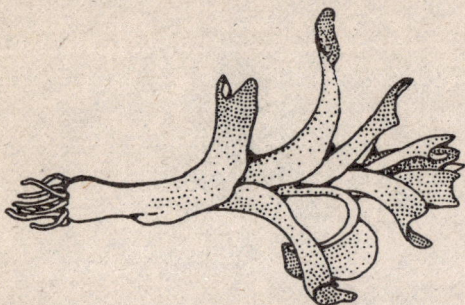

LEEK

Description: looks like a giant scallion.
Season: October–April.
Look for: smallish, long white root end.
Avoid: yellow or brown, spread, wilted, flower stalk.
Store: refrigerate.
Tip: rinse thoroughly to remove sand.

LETTUCE

Season: all year, best in spring and fall.

Crisp-Head (Iceberg)—the most common, rather tasteless.
Look for: heavy and firm, brittle leaves, green outside.
Avoid: rust, large root.

Butterhead (Boston, Bibb)—soft, flexible leaves, delicate, delicious.
Look for: dark green outside, white inside, heavy.
Avoid: wilted, bruised (especially Bibb).

Romaine or Cos—long head, long, narrow leaves, sweet tasting.
Look for: dark green, whitish near the root, crisp.
Avoid: wilted, deadened edges.

Leaf—loose leaves, highly perishable, tasty.
Look for: crisp, pleasant green (Red Leaf variety tinged with dark red).
Avoid: wilted, deadened edges.

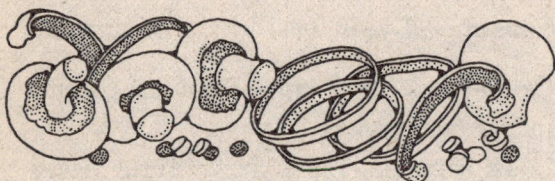

MUSHROOMS
Cultivated—the ordinary white mushroom.
Season: all year.
Look for: small, caps close to the stems, firm, plump.
Avoid: caps open with gills showing, dark gills, bruised.

Boletus—more often known as Cepes (French), Porcini (Italian) or Shitake (Japanese).
Season: summer–fall.

Chanterelles—taste like a woodsy combination of pepper and apricot.
Season: summer–winter.

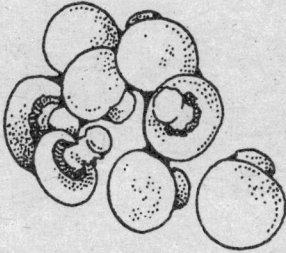

Shiitake—brown with beige marbling, meaty, earthy taste; woody stem is usually discarded before cooking.

Enoki—looks like a combination of bean sprouts and antennae.
Season: all year.
Look for: firm.
Avoid: soft, bruised.
Store: refrigerate in a shallow pan covered with a damp cloth.
Tip: for Chanterelles, put salt in a pan, cover tightly, and heat to disgorge water before final cooking.

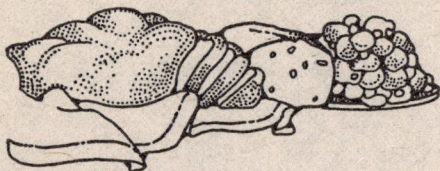

MUSTARD GREENS
Description: broad, flat, crinkle-edged leaves.
Season: all year.
Look for: crisp, rich green.
Avoid: wilted, yellow.
Store: refrigerate wrapped.

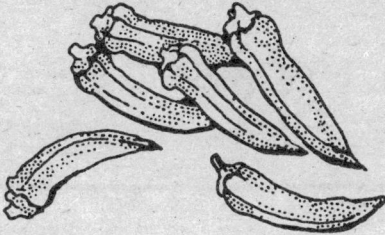

OKRA

Description: pointed green ridged fingers.
Season: all year.
Look for: small, flexible, green.
Avoid: large, stiff or soft, rust, pale.
Store: refrigerate wrapped.

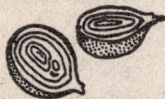

ONION

The names of the different varieties vary somewhat with region, but the following list should do:

Bermuda—flat, thick, mild.

Pearl—also called Pickling onions; tiny, usually peeled.

Shallots—tan with a hint of red and gray, the most subtle of flavors, and the highest status in the onion family.

Red—either oval (Italian) or round; pungent.

Spartan Sleeper—golden brown, round; will store at room temperature for months; good flavor.

Spanish—large, globe-shaped, white, yellow, or tan; sweet, mild and juicy.

Vidalia—looks like a flat yellow, unusually sweet, juicy and digestible.

White—bright white; the small ones are called Boiling onions.
Yellow—golden brown, globe-shaped, flat topped in the summer, very tasty.

Season: all year.
Look for: hard, firm, heavy, with dry skin like paper and slender flexible stems.
Avoid: wet, sprouting, green or black spots, soft, cracked.
Store: in a cool, dark, dry place, ventilated.
Tip: most of the tears come from the ends, so don't cut them.

Scallions—also called Spring or Green onions, they are young onions picked before the large bulb has formed.
Look for: crisp, faint blue to the green leaves.
Avoid: wilted, yellow, bruised.
Store: refrigerate wrapped.

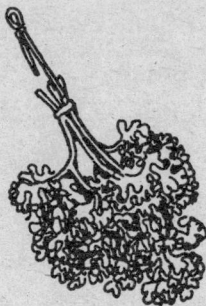

PARSLEY

Curly—more feathery than curly.

Italian—flat-leafed, more flavor.

Season: all year.

Look for: crisp, dark green.

Avoid: yellow or brown, moist, wilted, bruised.

Store: refrigerate or freeze wrapped.

Tips: • very nutritious, better eaten than used as decoration.

• said to be good antidote to garlic breath if eaten after serious garlic meal.

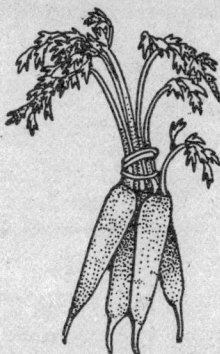

PARSNIP

Description: looks like a whitish-tan carrot.

Season: December–March.

Look for: small, firm, crisp, smooth.

Avoid: large, flabby, cracked, dry, discolored.

Store: refrigerate wrapped.

Tips: • peel after cooking.
   • tastes great roasted.

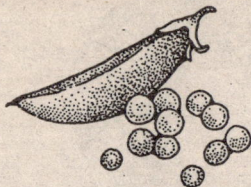

PEAS

Garden—the standard; includes Petits Pois, small-seeded peas picked very young.
Season: March–June.
Snow Peas—like its other name, Mange-Tout, you eat it pod and all; popular in Chinese dishes.
Season: all year.

Sugar Snap—sweet peas with edible pods; an excellent combination of the characteristics of both Garden and Snow.
Season: all year.

Look for: bright green, shiny, crisp, velvet pods.
Avoid: dull, yellow, limp.
Store: refrigerate one day maximum.

PEPPER

Hot—there is a bewildering variety, with names changing with each region. Generally, the smaller the hotter, but it is best to ask.

Sweet:

Green—the familiar Bell pepper.

Italian—pale green, elongated and contorted, more flavor than the Green or Red.

Red—a mature Green, slightly sweeter.

Yellow—similar to Green but milder and sweeter.

Season: all year, best March–December.

Look for: firm, crisp, rich color.

Avoid: soft, water spots, cracked, bruised.

Store: refrigerate in an airtight container.

Tip: to store peppers longer, remove the core and seeds.

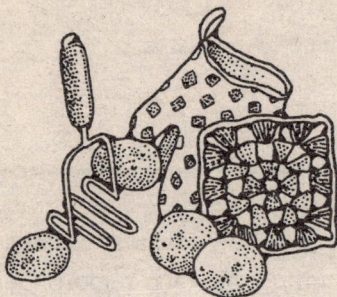

POTATO

Russet—sometimes called Idaho, despite also coming from other places; large and long with rough skin; for baking especially.

Red—small, round, red, smooth skinned, and very tasty, also called Red Bliss.

Round White—small, round, white, all-purpose.

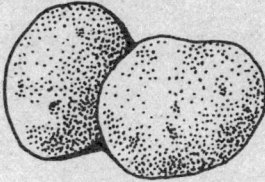

Long White—large, long, white, all-purpose.
New—Not a specific variety, but any potato picked early, usually the Reds and Whites.

Season: all year.
Look for: firm, smooth, evenly shaped.
Avoid: cuts, bruises, green, soft spots, sprouting.
Store: in a cool, dark, well-ventilated place.
Tips: • to keep them from turning black after peeling, place them in water.
• Do not eat if you see any green on the skin.

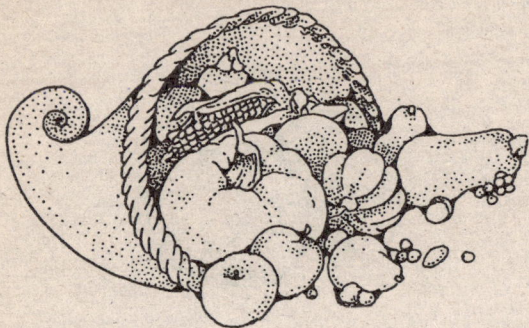

PUMPKIN

Season: October–November.

Look for: firm, heavy, bright skin.

Avoid: soft, lightweight, dull, cracked, discolored.

Store: in a cool, dark, dry place.

Tips: • roasted seeds are tasty too.

• tastiest pumpkins are small and firm.

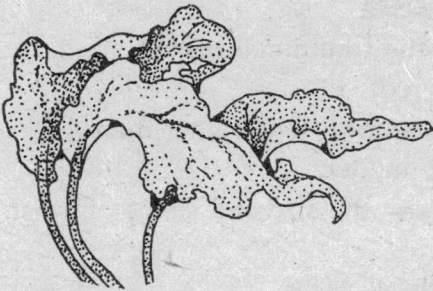

RABE

Description: spiky green leaves on stem, looks like dandelions.

Season: November–March.

Look for: bright green, crisp.

Avoid: yellow, wilted, insect holes.

RADISH

Red—the traditional marble-sized bright red.
White—small, long rather than round, milder.
Chinese—the size and shape of a fist.

Season: all year.
Look for: firm, glossy, bright, small in summer, medium in winter.
Avoid: cracked, flabby, wilted tops.
Store: remove tops, refrigerate.

RUTABAGA

Description: round, tan, hard, larger than a fist, usually waxed.
Season: October–December.
Look for: smooth, firm, small, heavy, yellow.
Avoid: cracked, sprouting, blemished.
Store: in a cool, dark, dry, well-ventilated place.

94

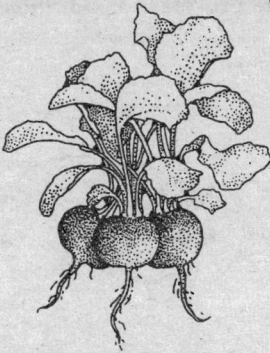

SPINACH

Season: all year.

Look for: crisp, dark green, small leaves.

Avoid: yellow, bruised, wilted.

Store: refrigerate in plastic.

Tip: wash carefully to remove grit.

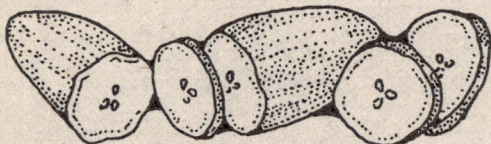

SQUASH (SUMMER)

Cocozelle—elongated, dark green with lighter green stripes, quite small, any size.

Patty Pan—also called Scallop, disk-shaped, green to white, about 3–4 inches across maximum.

Yellow Crookneck—small, yellow, almost pear-shaped, with a slender crooked neck, 4–5 inches maximum.

Yellow Straightneck—small, yellow, almost pear-shaped, with a slender straight neck, 4–5 inches maximum.

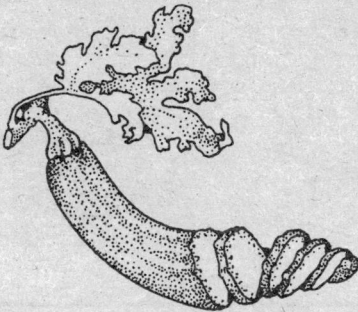

Zucchini—slender, elongated, dark green, 8–9 inches maximum.

Season: all year.
Look for: heavy, firm but tender, glossy, no larger than sizes listed above.
Avoid: dull, soft spots, dry, tough, flabby, mold.
Store: refrigerate.

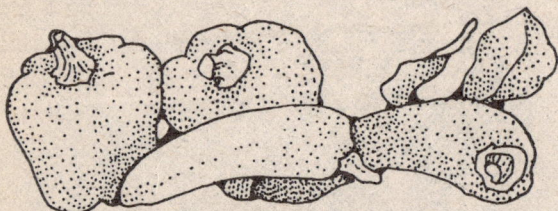

SQUASH (WINTER)

Acorn—aptly named, dark green, 5–6 inches, the most common variety, usually baked.

Boston Marrow—red-orange, about 15 pounds, perhaps the most beautiful, frequently baked.

Buttercup—large green stripes on green, 5–6 inches, similar to Acorn inside.

Butternut—yellow, pear-shaped, 1–3 pounds, perhaps the finest flavor.

Cushaw—golden or white with green stripes, up to 10 pounds.

Delicious—red-orange, 10–15 pounds, beautiful and tasty.

Golden Acorn—bright yellow, up

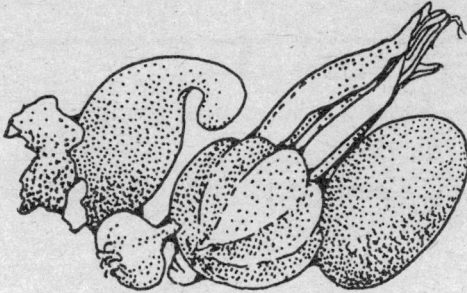

to 5 inches; when young can be eaten raw.

Hubbard—various colors, huge, over 15 pounds, beautiful and tasty.

Spaghetti—yellow, over 4 pounds; when cooked the flesh is scooped out and looks like spaghetti.

Turban—multicolored, really looks like a turban, delightful to look at and good to eat.

Season: October–December; all year for Acorn.

Look for: heavy, tough, hard.

Avoid: soft spots, cracks, mold, dull color.

Store: anywhere that's cool, dark, and dry, though a refrigerator will do.

99

SWEET POTATO

Moist—usually called yams; orange, sweet, delicious.

Dry—light peach color, dry grainy flesh.

Season: September–January.

Look for: firm, even color, smooth skin, small.

Avoid: soft spots, shriveled ends, sunken areas.

Store: dry, dark, well-ventilated, cool (but not the refrigerator).

Tip: True yams are never seen in this country, so you can keep calling sweet potatoes yams if you like.

SWISS CHARD

Description: broad, crinkled green leaves.

Season: November–March.

100

Look for: bright green, crisp.
Avoid: yellow, wilted, insect holes.
Store: refrigerate wrapped.
Tips: use like spinach, raw or cooked.

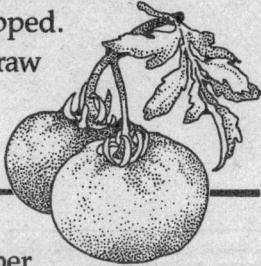

TOMATO

Season: June–September.
Look for: fragrant, firm but tender, plump, rich color.
Avoid: bruised, water spots, cracked, soft, hard (except green cooking tomatoes).
Store: ripen at room temperature, then refrigerate.
Tips: Out-of-season tomatoes are cold stored (making ripening impossible) and ethylene gassed into the appearance of ripeness and the aroma, taste, and texture of a football. Wait for the summer to feast on your local variety, and eat something else from October to May.

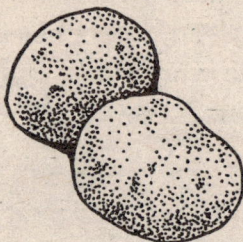

TRUFFLES

White—also called Alba or Piedmontese, looks a bit like a small potato; the best among truffles; usually grated uncooked onto dishes.

Black—also called Perigord, looks like a small black rock; perhaps not as good as the White, but not chopped liver either; always cooked.

Morel—usually looks like a dried-up sponge, sometimes thought to be a mushroom; a smoky flavor.

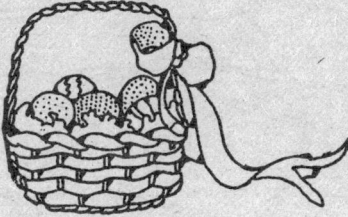

Season: November–February.
Look for: firm, dusty, full-looking.
Avoid: very hard or soft, wet spots, slimy.
Store: refrigerate in a closed container buried in rice (to absorb moisture).

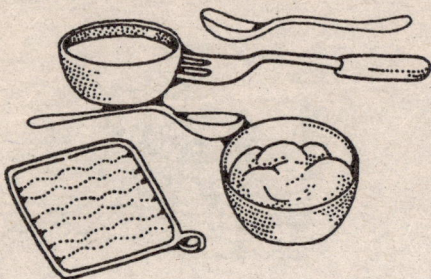

TURNIP

Description: round, firm, red or purple on top, white on bottom, smaller than a fist.

Season: March–May is best; also available October–December.

Look for: smooth, firm, small, heavy, white.

Avoid: cracked, sprouting, blemished.

Store: refrigerate.

Tip: very good in soup, stews, roasted.

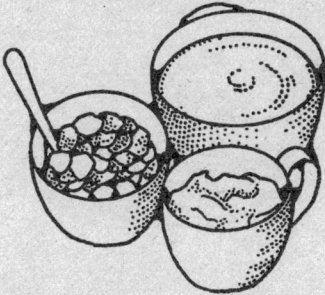

WATER CHESTNUT

Description: looks like dried-up chestnuts; crunchy.

Season: all year.

Look for: firm.

Avoid: soft, cracked, mold.

Store: in a cool, dark, dry, well-ventilated place.

Tip: look in Oriental markets.

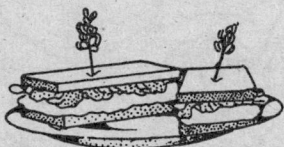

WATERCRESS

Description: a small green plant with somewhat triangular leaves at the end of the stem.

Season: all year.

Look for: crisp, rich green.

Avoid: yellow, wilted.

Store: refrigerate carefully wrapped.

Tip: use as soon as possible.

Meat

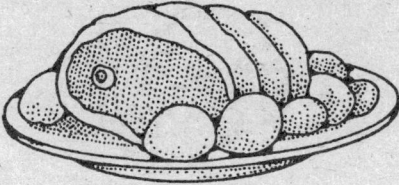

The most useful thing you can do to improve your meat shopping is to talk to your butcher, even if you shop in a supermarket. His knowledge and advice, as well as his goodwill, will get you safer and better quality meat for less money. He probably also knows how to cook it and wants to tell you. Regulation, inspection, and what goes into the meat we eat all remain controversial after almost a century of reporting. The assurance of a person you talk to every week has not lost its merit.

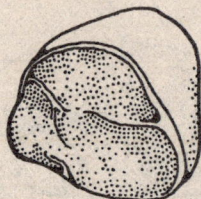

CHOOSING

Look for:
Beef—white fat, cherry-red meat, velvet texture.
Lamb and Veal—porous red bones.
Pork—light pink, firm, fine grain.
Circular inspection stamp which says,
"U.S. INSP'D & P'S'D."
Avoid: torn packaging, not refrigerated. A quantity of blood in the package indicates sitting out too long.
beef—yellow fat and dark meat.
lamb and veal—white flinty bones.

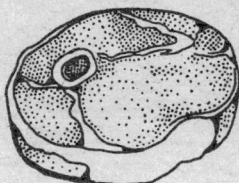

Beef, veal, and lamb are all cut up in a similar way—into seven sections you would expect to find on any mammal:

arm
shoulder blade
breast
rib
loin
hip
leg

All the roasts and steaks and chops and whatnot are based on these seven, and when organized this way (as they are in this chapter), they are a bit easier to keep track of. Pork is only slightly different.

111

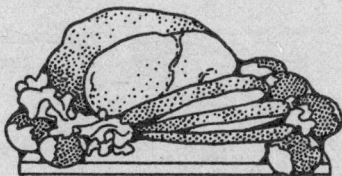

STORING

Refrigerator:
Wrapping: loose so air can circulate; remove original wrapper, rewrap.
Temperature: 35–40°.
Time:
Roasts and steaks: 3–5 days.
Chops, ground, stew, variety: 1–2 days.

Freezer:
Wrapping: tight to keep out air and moisture. wrap tight in moisture-proof freezer paper. Write both contents and date on package (you won't remember.)

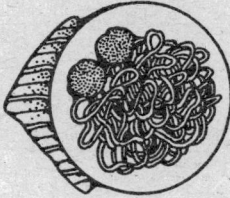

Temperature: 0° Fahrenheit (buy a thermometer).

Time: This is the maximum before both flavor and tenderness begin to deteriorate. For every 10° above 0°, the maximum is half as long.

Ground and stew: 2–4 months.

Beef: 8–12 months.

Veal: 4–8 months.

Pork:

Chops: 3–4 months.

Roasts: 4–8 months.

Sausage: 1–2 months.

Ham: 1–2 months.

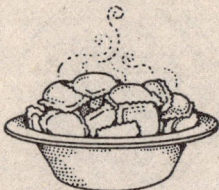

Lamb:
> *Chops:* 3–4 months.
> *Roasts:* 4–8 months.

Any smoked (cured) meat, including sausage, should not be frozen more than 2–4 months, because after that the salt added in curing turns the fat rancid.

To avoid the possibility of food poisoning:
Freeze as soon as possible after buying.
Do not refreeze meat once it has thawed completely.
Do not thaw in hot water.

Tip: Buying meat in bulk is not likely to be a savings. It may be more expensive,

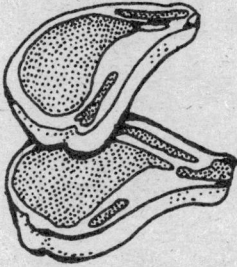

and you may not get the quality of meat you are used to. Dishonest advertising, hustling, and other lapses in integrity are not unheard of. However, buying large roasts, chucks, and bottom rounds when they are on sale and then cutting them yourself is an excellent way to save.

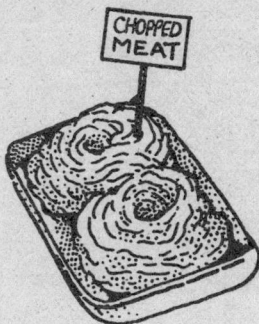

BEEF

Quality grade: Firm fat well distributed is called marbling, giving taste and tenderness. The more marbling, the higher the grade.

Look for shield inspection stamp:
USDA PRIME: restaurants; retail grade with the most marbling and (since that means the most fat) the most wasteful.
USDA CHOICE: the most often seen retail grade with the most marbling.
USDA GOOD: retail; not as tasty and tender as choice but more protein per pound and per dollar.

116

USDA STANDARD: seldom sold retail; a young animal, tender but not tasty.

USDA COMMERCIAL: frankfurters, sausages, cold cuts.

USDA UTILITY
USDA CUTTER } processed meats, animal food.
USDA CANNER

Yield grade: You will seldom see this on trimmed meat. It is the percentage of meat in relation to bone and fat; numbered 1 (the most meat) to 5.

Beef is aged by hanging it for two to eight weeks at 34°–38° to let the natural bacterial process break down the meat's connective tissues. The trimming of the resultant discoloration together with all this storage is of course costly. Whether or not it makes the meat better is debatable. Various other methods have been devised to save time and waste less meat, and therefore cost less, but they have yet to become universally popular.

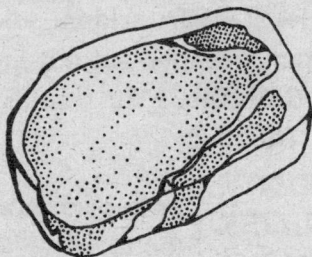

Beef Cuts

ARM:

**Center Beef Shanks or
    Shank Cross-cuts**—braise or cook in
    liquid.

Stew Meat—braise or cook in liquid.

SHOULDER BLADE (CHUCK):

Stew Meat—braise or cook in liquid.

Neck or Yankee Pot Roast—braise or cook
    in liquid.

Beef Neck Bones—cook in liquid.

Boneless Pot Roast—braise.

Beef Chuck Pot Roast—braise.

Chuck Roast Blade Cut—braise or roast.

Top Chuck Roast—braise.

Bottom Chuck Roast—braise or roast.

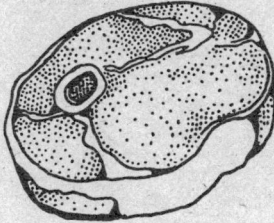

**Boneless Roast or
  Boneless Chuck Roast**—braise or roast.
Boneless Chuck Steak—braise, broil, or
  fry.
Chuck Fillet—braise.
**Chicken Steak or
  Top Chuck Steak, Boneless**—braise or
  fry.
**Boneless Chuck Fillet or
  Chuck Eye Roast, Boneless**—braise or
  roast.
Cross-Rib Roast—braise.
Knuckle Bone Soup Bone—cook in liquid.
Ribs, Barbecue
     Braising
     Short

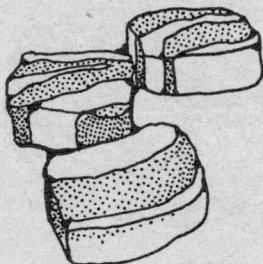

Chuck Short
Kosher—braise or cook in liquid.

Beef Chuck Shoulder Steak, Boneless—braise.

Shoulder Roast, Boneless—braise.

BREAST:

Brisket—braise or cook in liquid.

Boneless Brisket—braise or cook in liquid.

RIB:

**Beef Rib Pot Roast or
Standing Rib Roast**—roast.

Rib Steak—broil or fry.

**Delmonico or
Rib Eye**—broil or fry.

Rib Eye Roast—roast.

Short Ribs—braise or cook in liquid.

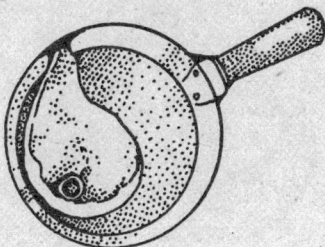

**Flank Steak or
  London Broil**—braise or broil.
Flank Steak, Cubed—braise, broil, or fry.
Ground Beef (Hamburger)—braise, broil,
  or fry.
Cubed Steak—braise, broil, or fry.
**Rolled Beef Plate or
  Yankee Pot Roast**—braise.
LOIN (SHORT LOIN):
**Club Steak,
  Shell Steak, or
  Sirloin Strip Steak**—braise, broil, or fry.
**Kansas City Steak,
  New York Strip Steak, or
  Boneless Club Sirloin Steak**—broil or
  fry.

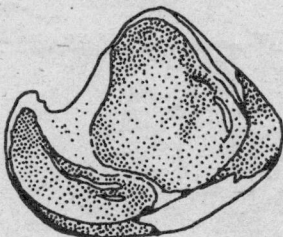

T-Bone—broil or fry.
Porterhouse Steak—broil or fry.
Tenderloin Roast,
   Filet Mignon Roast, or
   Chateaubriand—roast or broil.
Beef Fillet Steak or
   Filet Mignon—broil or fry.
HIP:
Sirloin Steak, round bone (the best)
                  pin bone
                  flat bone
                  wedge bone and boneless—
                     broil or fry.
LEG:
Rump Roast—braise or roast.
Boneless Rump Roast—braise or roast.

122

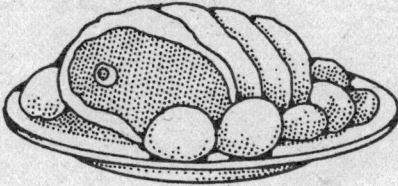

**Top Round Steak, Center Cut or
  (cut very thin) Bracciole**—broil or fry.
**Cubed Steak or
  Minute Steak**—braise or fry.
**Bottom Round or
  Bottom Round Pot Roast**—braise or
  roast.
Eye Round Roast—braise or roast.
Eye Round Steak—braise, broil, or fry.
**Sirloin Tip Roast or
  Round Tip Roast**—braise or roast.
Trimmed Sirloin Tip Roast—braise or roast.
Sirloin Tip Steak—broil or fry.
Beef Kabobs—braise or broil.
Beef Heel Pot Roast—braise or cook in
  liquid.

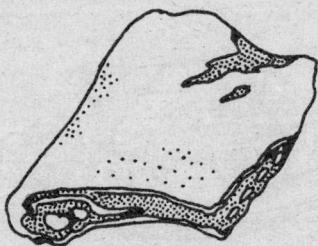

VEAL

Veal is both a good buy and probably healthier than other meats. Since it contains less fat, less fat is wasted and less fat gets into your bloodstream. And since it is slaughtered young, it has had far less exposure to the drugs and hormones cattle receive.

Quality grades for retail are the same as for beef.

ARM:
Veal Shank Cross-cuts—braise or cook in liquid.

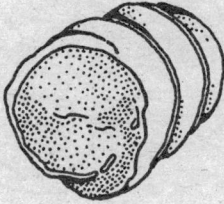

SHOULDER BLADE:
Veal Stew or
  Veal Stew, Boneless—braise or cook in liquid
Veal Shoulder Roast—braise or roast.
Shoulder or
  Shoulder Chops—braise or fry.
Rolled Veal Roast—braise or roast.
Veal Shoulder, Roast—braise or roast.
Veal Chops—braise or fry.
Veal Rib Roast—roast.

BREAST:
Breast of Veal—braise or roast.
Riblets—braise or cook in liquid.

RIB:
Veal Rib Roast—roast.
Veal Rib Chops—braise or fry.

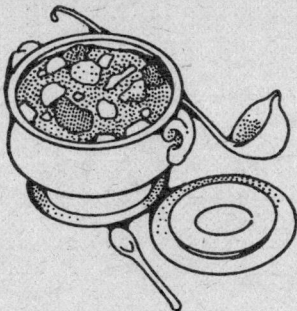

LOIN:

Veal Loin Roast—roast.

Veal Kidney Chops—braise or fry.

HIP:

Veal Sirloin Roast—braise or fry.

Veal Sirloin Chop—braise or fry.

Rolled Double Sirloin—braise or fry.

LEG:

Rump Roast—braise or roast.

Rolled Rump Roast—braise or roast.

Leg of Veal—braise or roast.

Veal Scallopini—braise or fry.

Heel Round Roast—braise or fry.

Veal Cubed Steak—braise or fry.

Veal Stew—braise.

Veal Cutlets—braise or fry.

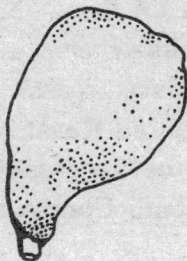

LAMB

Quality grades for retail are the same as for beef.

If you want to avoid chemical treatment of the animals you will eat, New Zealand lamb is free from hormones, tenderizers, and tranquilizers. It is of course frozen for shipping to this country.

Lamb Cuts

ARM:
Lamb Shank—braise or cool in liquid.
SHOULDER BLADE:
Stewing Lamb—braise or broil.

Lamb Neck for Stew—braise.

Shish Kebobs—braise.

Shoulder Roast—roast.

**Boneless Rolled Roast or
    Rolled Shoulder Roast**—roast.

Shoulder Lamb Chop—braise, broil, or
    fry.

Lamb Shank—braise or cook in liquid.

BREAST:

Breast of Lamb—braise or roast.

**Riblets or
    Lamb Breast Riblets**—braise or roast.

Lamb Spareribs—braise, broil, or roast.

RIB:

**Lamb Rib Rack or
    Lamb Rack Roast**—roast.

Rib Lamb Chops—braise, broil, or fry.

Lamb Patties—braise, broil, or fry.

LOIN:
Saddle Roast or
  Lamb Loin Roast—roast.
Double Chops or
  English Lamb Chops—broil or fry.
Loin Chops—broil or fry.
HIP:
Sirloin Chops—broil or fry.
Sirloin Roast—roast.
LEG:
Leg of Lamb—roast.
Boneless Lamb Leg—roast.
Lamb Leg, Center Slice—broil or fry.
Lamb Leg, French Style—roast.
American Leg—roast.
Cube Lamb Steaks—broil or fry.
Leg of Lamb, Butt Half or
  Sirloin Half—roast.
Leg of Lamb, Shank Half—roast.

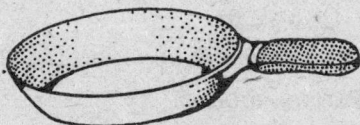

PORK

Quality grades: 1, 2, and 3, describing only the amount of fat on animal.

Pork Cuts

JOWL:
Smoked Pork Jowl—whole: cook in liquid.
   sliced: cook in liquid or broil.

ARM:
Pork Hock or
   Pork Shank—braise or cook in liquid.
Pork Shoulder Arm Roast—roast.
Pig's Feet—braise or cook in liquid.
Pork Shoulder Arm Picnic—braise, broil, or fry.

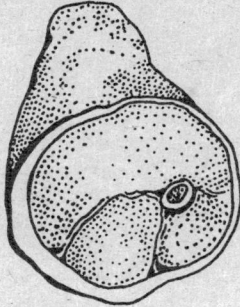

**Smoked Pork Shoulder Roll or
  Smoked Picnic**—bake, roast, or cook in
  liquid.
Arm Steak—braise or fry.
**Pork Hock or
  Pork Shank**—braise or cook in liquid.
**SHOULDER (CALLED BOSTON
  SHOULDER):**
**Pork Butt or
  Boneless Rolled Pork Butt**—roast.
Pork Shoulder Blade Steak—braise, broil,
  or fry.
Fat Back—fry or cook in liquid.
RIB:
Spareribs—bake, roast, broil, or cook in
  liquid.

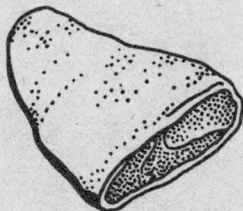

Fresh Side of Pork—cook in liquid.

Bacon (same as above, smoked)—fry or broil.

LOIN:

**Pork Loin or
    Rib End Roast**—roast.

Rib End Pork Chops—braise, broil, or fry.

**Country Style Spareribs or
    Country Ribs**—braise, bake, roast, or cook in liquid.

**Pork Barbecue Ribs or
    Pork Loin Back Ribs**—braise, bake, roast, or cook in liquid.

Pork Loin Center Rib Roast—roast.

Center Cut Pork Chops—braise, broil, or fry.

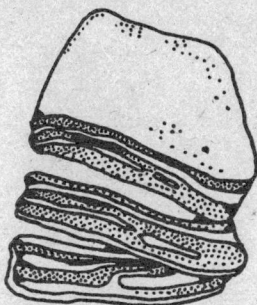

Boneless Pork Loin Roast—roast.
Canadian Bacon—braise, broil, or fry.
LEG:
Fresh Ham or Pork Leg, Whole.
Butt Half Fresh Ham or Pork Leg, Sirloin Half or Rump Half.
Shank Half Fresh Ham or Pork Leg, Shank Half.

For all three of the above,
if fresh: roast,
if smoked: roast,
if smoked and cooked ("ready to eat"): eat.

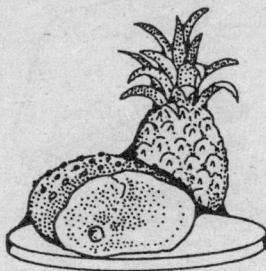

VARIETY MEATS

These meats are highest in B vitamins, iron, and protein, or in other words, the things we eat meat for. They are also relatively low in calories.

Brains—tender, very tasty, cook as soon as possible or precook in liquid.

Heart—not very tender but very tasty. Beef is the largest and least tender and requires the longest cooking. Veal is the most delicate but much smaller. Roast with fat tied around the surface.

Liver—extraordinary nutritive value. Do not overcook.

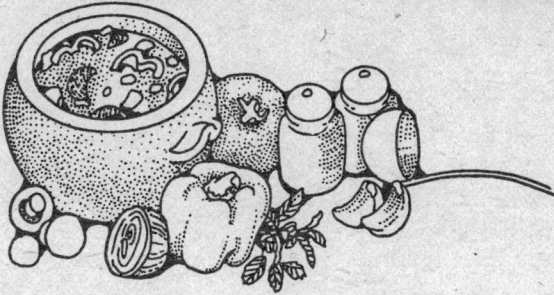

Calf—the most delicate; broil or fry.
Beef—not as tender but cheaper; braise or fry.
Pork—most flavorful, least tender; braise.
Kidney—remove membrane and inside part on bottom if necessary.
Lamb, Veal—broil, fry, or cook in liquid.
Pork, Beef—braise or cook in liquid.
Tongue—very tasty, requires long cooking in water.
Oxtails—good in soups and stews, or cooked on their own in water for a long time.

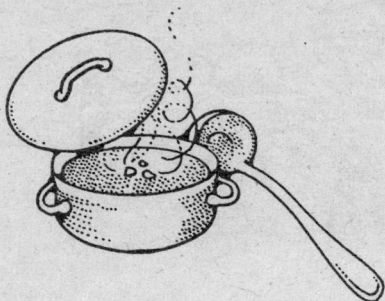

Tripe—the inner lining of beef stomach; three kinds: honeycomb
pocket
plain.

Requires long cooking in water, then braise, fry, or broil.

Sweetbreads—look for reddish color, bright. Precook in water 25 minutes, then braise, broil, or fry.

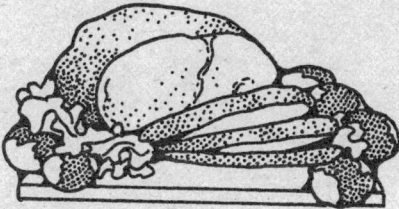

OTHER ANIMALS
Mutton
Meat from the sheep, or, from the consumer's point of view, an old lamb.

Under 1 year—still a lamb.
1–2 years—yearling mutton.
Over 2 years—mutton.

Quality grades are the same as lamb without a Prime grade. The bone at the foot joint is hard and white; a lamb's is still porous, moist, and reddish.

Venison
Generally, any animal from the deer family, all of which is kosher. Unless the

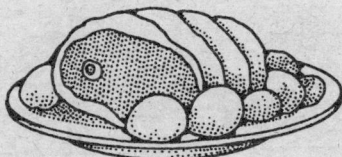

animal is very young, it must be hung and marinated before eating. When young, venison may be broiled or grilled or even roasted larded with pork fat.

Look for: moist, velvety, clean fresh smell.
Avoid: not wet.
Cuts: haunch, loin, or fillets.

Rabbit
Light, delicate meat similar to chicken.
Look for: moist, flesh springy to the touch, fresh pink color, smell good, dark red liver.
Avoid: liver splotched with white.

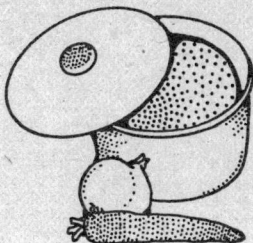

Snails (Escargots)
They must be alive if they aren't canned.

Frog's Legs
Look for: springy, pale pink, pleasant smell.

Poultry

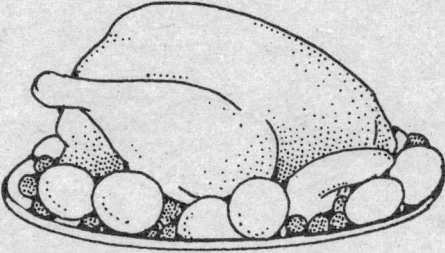

Poultry is inspected for wholesomeness and stamped by the USDA, though you may not find the stamp very easily.

Quality grades are A, B, and C, corresponding to Prime, Choice, and Good in other meats. Unlike other meats, however, the grade does not refer to tenderness. Grade A means the bird is attractive and meaty.

The bird's age determines tenderness.

Look for: plump breasts and legs, short legs, soft, moist, smooth, yellow to cream color, few pinfeathers. The breastbones in chickens and turkeys and the bills in ducks and geese should be flexible if the bird is

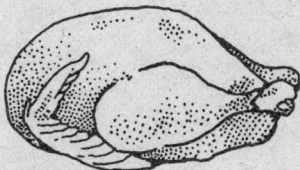

young. Ducks should always have flat, wide breasts and plump backs.

Avoid: wet or dry, bluish skin, scaly or brittle legs, unpleasant odor.

Store: refrigerate loosely wrapped or freeze tightly wrapped. Remove all stuffing from bird before refrigerating after it's cooked.

To avoid the possibility of food poisoning:
Keep the bird cold while preparing it for storage (cutting, wrapping, etc.).
Do not refreeze if bird has thawed completely.
Wash all utensils, containers, cutting boards, and hands thoroughly before they touch anything else.

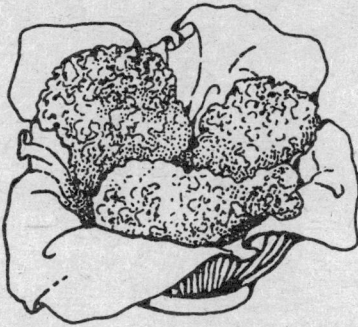

All frozen birds should be thawed in the refrigerator. Do not thaw in hot water. Turkeys come with their own instructions.

Tip: Chicken and turkey make a cheap substitute for veal cutlets.

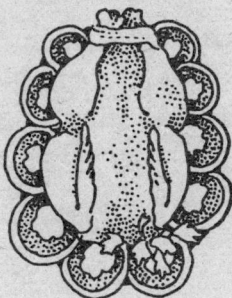

CHICKEN

Squab Chicken—a 1-pound baby bird.

Broiler-Fryer—7–9 weeks, 1½–3½ pounds, extremely tender; 90 percent of all chickens sold can be cooked in any way.

Roaster—12–16 weeks, 3½–7 pounds, quite plump.

Capon—under 8 months, 4–7 pounds, a castrated male, extra white meat.

Fowl or Heavy Hen or Stewing Chicken—a hen over 10 months old, 4½–6 pounds, tough, good for soup.

TURKEY

Fryer-Roaster—under 16 weeks, 4–9 pounds.

Young Hen, Young Tom—5–7 months, 10–25 pounds, best roasted.

Yearling Hen, Young Tom—over 1 year, 10–25 pounds, best roasted.

Mature Hen, Mature Tom—over 15 months, 10–25 pounds, best ignored.

Turkeys can be: small—4–10 pounds.
medium—10–19 pounds.
large—over 20 pounds.

Butterball is a self-basting turkey because 3 per cent of its fat is coconut oil (a saturated fat) and water which have been injected into it. As this excess fat cooks it rises to the surface and bastes the turkey.

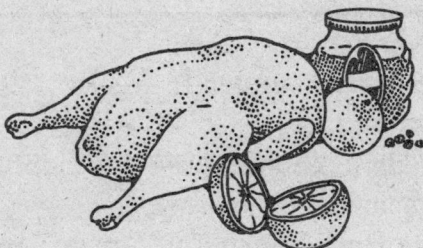

DUCK
Broiler or Fryer—under 8 weeks, 3 pounds.
Roaster Duckling—8–16 weeks, 3–7 pounds.

GOOSE
Under 11 months, 4–14 pounds, roast.

GUINEA HEN
Dry, gentle yet gamy, 2–4 pounds.

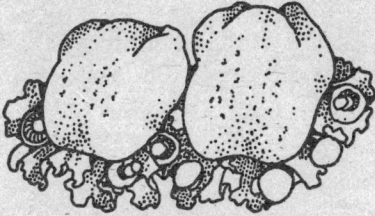

PHEASANT
Dry but tasty, 2–4 pounds.

ROCK CORNISH GAME HEN
A new breed of roasting chicken, about 1½ pounds, plump and tasty.

SQUAB
A pigeon raised for eating, about 1 pound.

Fish and Shellfish

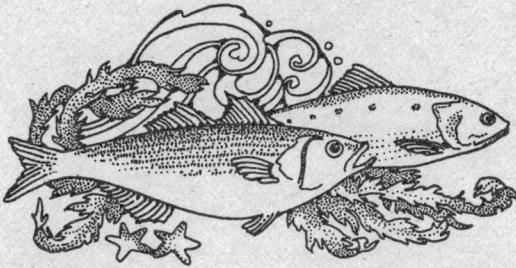

FISH

Inspection of fish and shellfish is entirely voluntary, and combined with their being extremely perishable and the disease-carrying propensities of shellfish, this makes for some pretty chancy shopping. With shellfish, it's impossible to know if it's carrying a bit of hepatitis or whatnot. With freshwater fish, well, they've been swimming in some of our rivers and streams, so there's no telling even what it is you hope they don't have. Saltwater fish, however, are one of the safer bets around. The ocean has so far resisted pollution enough to continue to provide a great variety of low-calorie, high-protein, organically grown meals.

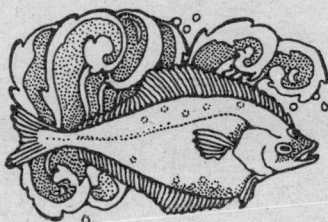

Look for: fish should be shipped and displayed on ice.

Whole—moist skin, shiny scales tight to the skin, bright, clear, protruding eyes, gills pink to red, fresh looking, flesh firm, should spring back when pressed with finger, no strong or unpleasant odor.

Pan-dressed: scaled, cleaned with head, tail, and fins removed.

Fillet: a side of fish, with or without the skin.

Steak: crosscut slice from large fish with skin and scales removed.

Fish sticks (not frozen fish sticks): 1-by-3-inch cuts.

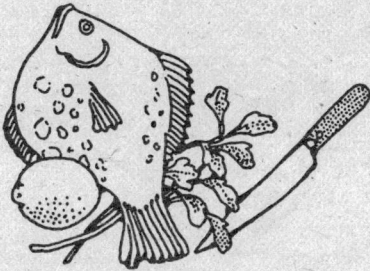

All four of these forms should have firm flesh and a sweet smell.

Avoid: cloudy, sunken eyes; slimy gills, faded skin.

Storage: eat as soon as possible. If necessary, wrap in foil or in covered dish; place in coldest part of refrigerator. To keep longer than a day or two, freeze it. Wrap tightly in moisture-proof paper, separating individual pieces with freezer paper.

To avoid the possibility of food poisoning:
 Fish that has been frozen and thawed should never be eaten raw.
 Keep cold while preparing for storage (cutting, wrapping, etc.).

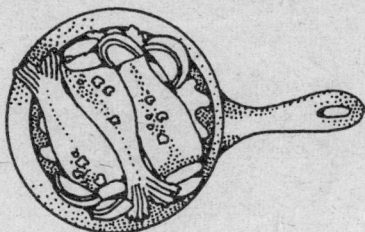

Do not refreeze fish once it has thawed completely.
Do not thaw in hot water; thaw in refrigerator.

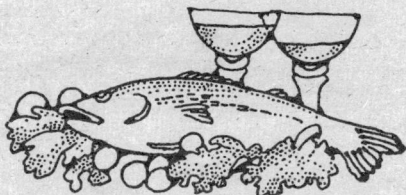

Saltwater Fish

Bluefish—fine grain, moist, dark flesh, lean.
Atlantic and Gulf

Butterfish—white, sweet, tender, fatty.
Atlantic and Gulf.

Cod—white, meaty, lean.
Atlantic and Pacific.

Croaker: delicate taste, lean.
Atlantic.

Drum (Channel Bass)—look for the less
bony red variety, lean.
Atlantic and Gulf.

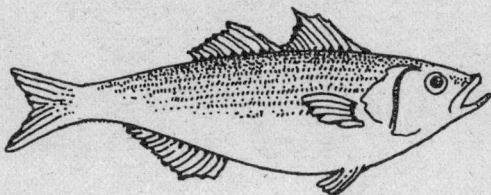

Eel—mild, finely textured, fatty.
Atlantic and Gulf.

Flounder—delicate, fine, white, lean,
sometimes called Lemon or Gray Sole.
Atlantic, Pacific, and Gulf.

Fluke (Plaice)—delicate, white, lean.
North Atlantic.

Haddock—fine grain, white, meaty, lean.
North Atlantic.

Halibut—large, flat, strong flavor, lean.
Atlantic and Pacific.

Herring—sardines (young Herring), shad,
and sprats are all related; fatty.
Atlantic and Pacific.

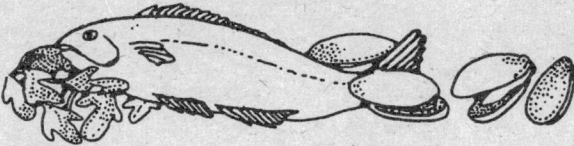

Kingfish—tasty, firm, fatty.
South Atlantic and Gulf.

Lingcod—delicate, white, lean.
Pacific.

Mackerel (Atlantic)—tasty, firm, strong
flavor, fatty.

Mackerel (Pacific)—tasty, firm, fatty, darker
than Atlantic.

Mullet—firm, strong flavor, fatty.
Atlantic and Gulf.

Ocean Perch—firm, white, flakes, subtle
flavor, lean.
North Atlantic.

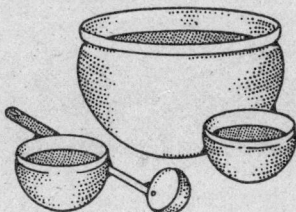

Pacific Sole—delicate, white, lean.
Pacific.

Pollack—like a firm, strong-flavored cod; lean.
North Atlantic.

Pompano—delicate, fine, and extraordinary.
South Atlantic and Gulf.

Porgy—tasty, white, lean.
Atlantic and Gulf.

Red Snapper—moist, mild and meaty, lean.
South Atlantic and Gulf.

Rockfish—mild, pink flesh, lean.
Pacific.

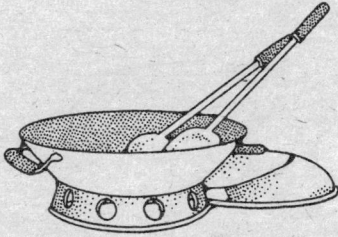

Sablefish—mild, white, tender, fatty.
Pacific.

Salmon—succulent, pink to orange, fatty.
North Atlantic and North Pacific.

Sea Bass—tasty if bony, moist, white, lean.
Atlantic.

Sea Squab (Blowfish)—pleasant and juicy,
lean.
Atlantic.

Shad—tasty and tender, white, fatty.
Atlantic and Pacific.

Shark—firm, meaty, fatty (frequently sold
as bogus scallops).
Atlantic and Pacific.

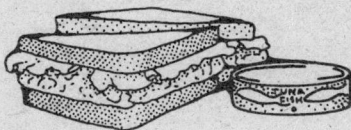

Skate—stingray wings, firm but gooey, lean. Atlantic and Pacific.

Smelt (Grunion, Whitebait)—tasty, firm, fatty.
Atlantic, Pacific, and Great Lakes.

Striped Bass—white, moist, lean.
Atlantic, Pacific, and Gulf.

Sturgeon—tasty, firm, lean.
North Atlantic, North Pacific.

Swordfish—firm, meaty, smoky, fatty.
South Atlantic, South Pacific.

Tautog (Blackfish)—lean meat, juicy.
Atlantic.

162

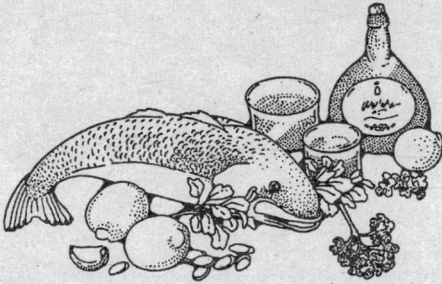

Tilefish—firm, meaty, mild (similar to Swordfish).
Atlantic and Gulf.

Tuna—strong flavor, firm, dark color, fatty.
Atlantic and Pacific.

Turbo—delicate, white, lean.
Atlantic and Pacific.

Weakfish—gentle flavor and texture, lean.
Atlantic and Gulf.

Whiting (Hake)—fine grain, mild flavor, white, lean.
North Atlantic.

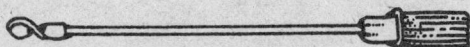

FRESHWATER FISH

Bass—very tasty, white, lean.
Entire U.S.

Carp—firm, often used for gefilte fish, fatty.
Entire U.S.

Catfish—rich flavor, firm, fatty.
East Coast to Rockies.

Muskellunge—bony with nice tender meat, lean.
East to Midwest.

Pickerel—bony with delicate flavor, lean.
East to Midwest.

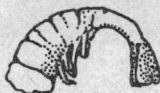

Pike—bony but tender, lean.
East to Midwest.

Salmon—much like the more famous saltwater salmon, fatty.
Northeast.

Sunfish (Bream)—very tasty, lean.
South to Midwest.

Trout—many varieties, all delicious, lean.
Entire U.S.

Whitefish—buttery, tasty, firm, fatty.
Northeast to Midwest.

Yellow Perch—small and tasty, lean.
East to Midwest and West.

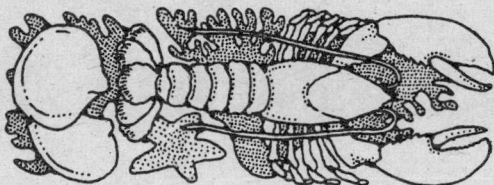

SHELLFISH

This is the most perishable of foods and requires care. The fresher the better. Shellfish should be juicy, with a delicate flavor. Most of the shellfish sold are already cooked, and too long at that, rendering them dry, tough, and tasteless. If you cook your own, you will probably be pleasantly surprised.

When bought uncooked: should be bought at last minute;
should be sold from the ice.

Avoid: damaged or partly open shells;
Never buy dead, raw shellfish in the shell.

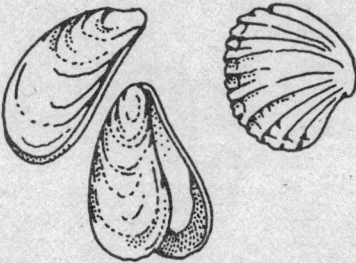

The dealer will usually prepare clams on the half shell for you.

ABALONE
Look for: tightly closed shells.

CLAMS
East Coast
Soft (Steamers)—also called Longnecks; long oval shape, black necks, ½–1 quart per person.
Hard Shell
  Chowder—3 inches or more, for chowder and stuffed clams.
  Cherrystone—2 inches, for steaming or half shell.
  Littleneck—1½ inches, for half shell.

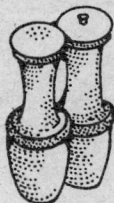

West Coast
Butter—small, sweet, for half shell.
Mud—large ovals from the north.
Pismo—at least 5 inches, sweet, very tender.
Razor—long, thin, and delicious, the clam de la clam.

Look for: tightly closed shells or shells that the clams themselves close at the tap of a finger.
Shucked clams—about 1 quart for four people.

Look for: plump, sweet smell.

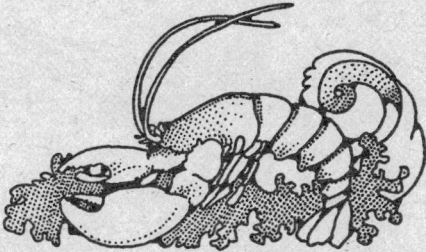

CONCH
Look for: the most recently docked boat. South Atlantic and Gulf.

CRAB
Alaska King—up to 6 feet and 20 pounds; only the leg meat is eaten.

Blue—the most popular.

Dungeness—big, pinkish-white, sweet, Pacific coast.

Rock—tan and tasty flesh.

Stone—a dish of claws, Florida.

Soft-shell crabs have merely shed their hard shell. In about 24 hours this too will harden, so they are quite expensive.

Look for: alive and kicking as much as possible.

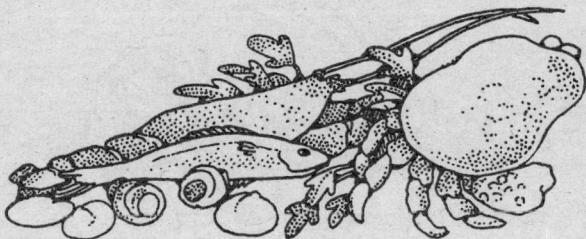

CRAYFISH

Looks like a pale, very small lobster.
Look for: alive and kicking as much as
possible.

LOBSTER

Look for: alive and downright active; tails
should curl back quickly when straightened.
The greener the better; half red is half
dead.

MUSSELS

Look for: tightly closed shells.
Tip: To clean, scrub with brush, cut off the
fiber on outside, and soak in cold water for
2 hours while they expel sand. Throw out
any mussels that float—they're dead.

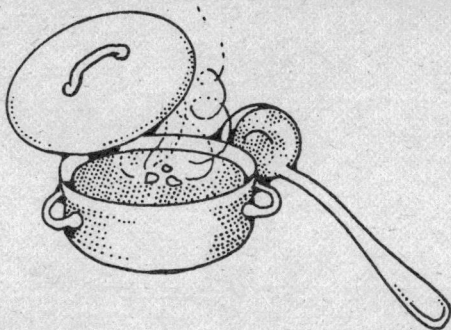

OCTOPUS
Look for: firm yet tender, pleasant smell, not too much liquid.

OYSTERS
Eastern
Blue Point—originally from Long Island.
Chincoteague—perhaps the great American oyster, from Virginia.

Western
Olympia—tiny and excellent.
Pacific (Japanese)—large, mostly fried.

Look for: tightly closed shells—either already shut or closing upon slight provocation.

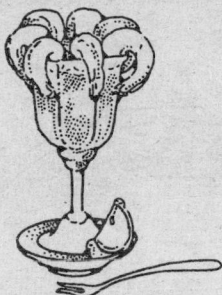

Shucked oysters should be cream-colored and plump.

SCALLOPS
Bay—tiny, pink to cream, very sweet.
Sea—an inch or more, tan, firm.
Look for: white to cream color, firm, sweet smell (even though strong).

SHRIMP
Colossal—less than 10 per pound.
Jumbo—10–15.
Medium—16–25.
Small—26–40.
Miniatures—over 200.

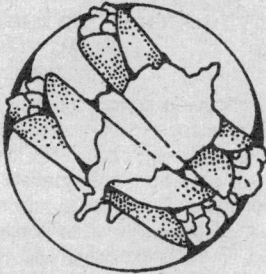

Look for: gray-green to tan, firm, moist, springy, sweet smell.

SQUID
Look for: firm yet tender, pleasant smell, not too much liquid.

TURTLE
Look for: springy, moist, rich color from white to green, even gray; the meat from the back is the best.

THE SMART SHOPPER

__LE GETTE'S GUIDE TO FRESH FOOD SHOPPING
by Bernard Le Gette   (M32-421, $2.95, U.S.A.)
                                (M32-422, $3.75, Canada)

This indispensable shopping companion guide is for today's economy-minded food shopper, who wants the highest quality available for the price. It is the only book of its kind on the market and will appeal to everyone from homemakers concerned with their families' nutrition to health fanatics to cooking enthusiasts—anyone who cares about the quality of the food they buy. Special features include tests for freshness, when and where to buy, and information on the different varieties of fresh food.

__THE UNDERGROUND SHOPPER'S GUIDE
TO OFF-PRICE SHOPPING   (M32-890, $4.50, U.S.A.)
by Sue Goldstein   (M32-891, $5.75, Canada)

How many people would like to buy name-brand merchandise at up to eighty percent off retail prices? According to *Advertising Age*, "Off-price shoppers are everywhere." Let this definitive reference book provide all the answers to the where, when, and how of bargain hunting anywhere in America. Find out about factory outlets, showrooms, discount trade shows, bartering, tips on recognizing knockoffs, and much, much more.

WARNER BOOKS
P.O. Box 690
New York, N.Y. 10019

Please send me the books I have checked. I enclose a check or money order (not cash), plus 50¢ per order and 50¢ per copy to cover postage and handling.* (Allow 4 weeks for delivery.)

_____ Please send me your free mail order catalog. (If ordering only the catalog, include a large self-addressed, stamped envelope.)

Name _____

Address _____

City _____

State _____ Zip _____

*N.Y. State and California residents add applicable sales tax.   127

From Very Famous Chefs

__BARBECUE WITH BEARD

James Beard   *(Z35-062, $2.75)*

This outdoor cookbook shows you how to turn out master-pieces every time. Every method of outdoor cooking is explored from a charcoal hibachi to an electric rotisserie. There are recipes for every main course from hamburgers to Chateaubriand—and for the accompaniments from dip to dessert. It's a gallery of good things to eat presented by the master himself.

__JAMES BEARD'S FISH COOKERY

James Beard   *(Z32-948, $4.95, U.S.A.)*
                                     (Z32-949, $6.25, Canada)

From halibut and salmon to grunion and pompano, trout to buffalo fish, or abalone to conch and oysters: James Beard has all the valuable information about how to choose and cook fish. Hundreds of delicious recipes makes this "a must for any good cook's collection."   —*Dallas Times Herald*

__MAIDA HEATTER'S BOOK OF GREAT DESSERTS

Maida Heatter   *(Z30-710, $4.95)*

Maida Heatter brings you her very best recipes in this book. From the easy-to-make Raspberry Strawberry Bavarian to the super-sophisticated Dobosh Torte, each recipe is accompanied by clear, step-by-step directions to insure that each comes out exactly as it should. Nothing is left vague. She tells you exactly where the racks should be placed in the oven, when and how to test, at what speed to set the electric beater—even how to improvise, if you must.

WARNER BOOKS
P.O. Box 690
New York, N.Y. 10019

Please send me the books I have checked. I enclose a check or money order (not cash), plus 50¢ per order and 50¢ per copy to cover postage and handling.* (Allow 4 weeks for delivery.)

_____ Please send me your free mail order catalog. (If ordering only the catalog, include a large self-addressed, stamped envelope.)

Name _____

Address _____

City _____

State _____ Zip _____

*N.Y. State and California residents add applicable sales tax.   87

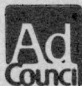